REGIONAL

GUIDE TO

HUMAN

ANATOMY

# REGIONAL GUIDE TO HUMAN ANATOMY

**Alan Twietmeyer, Ph.D.**
Associate Professor and Chairman
Division of Physical Education
Concordia College
Ann Arbor, Michigan
(formerly of Colorado State University)


**Thomas McCracken, M.S.**
Office of Biomedical Media and
Department of Anatomy
Colorado State University
Fort Collins, Colorado

Lea & Febiger  Philadelphia
1988

Lea & Febiger
600 South Washington Square
Philadelphia, PA  19106-4198
U.S.A.
(215) 922-1330

**Library of Congress Cataloging-in-Publication Data**

Twietmeyer, Alan.
  Regional guide to human anatomy.

  1. Anatomy, Surgical and topographical—
Outlines, syllabi, etc.  I. McCracken, Thomas.
II. Title.  [DNLM: 1. Anatomy, Regional.
QS 4 T972r]
QM531.T85  1988      611'.9  87-16944
ISBN 0-8121-1103-6

Printed in the United States of America

Print Number:  5 4 3 2 1

*To my loving and patient wife, Patricia, and our seven wonderful children: Geoffry, Andrew, Greggory, Julie, Jennifer, Janell and Nathanael*


*To my son, Sean, who put up with me during this endeavor*

# PREFACE

## GOAL

The goal of this guide/workbook is to provide students with a conceptual format for the study of gross human anatomy. The outline format and minimal text allows the student and instructor to work together in deciding which portions to include or exclude, thus allowing this book to be used in a variety of course levels. The authors feel that introductory human anatomy courses often do a disservice to the students by concentrating on specific facts while ignoring the conceptual picture and by not linking such concepts to the students' career objectives.

## AUDIENCE

Because of its modified outline approach this book is not self limiting to courses taught to certain groups of students or courses taught with or without laboratories. The most obvious audience includes students in allied health fields: physical education, occupational therapy, physical therapy, and athletic training or majors in biology, zoology, or art. However, enough factual information is presented in an easily accessible manner for this book to be an appropriate review source for students in medicine, dentistry, and nursing.

## APPROACH AND RATIONALE

Two approaches are interwoven in this guide. One is the approach of presenting material regionally. The authors believe that such an approach aids the student in creating an understanding of the interrelationship of anatomic structures.

The second approach is one of doing. The illustrations are provided with identifying letters or numbers in accordance with the outline, but the student should label these. Other structures associated with a particular illustration may also be labelled by the learner. The authors encourage any active participation such as coloring and notation. In addition many opportunities are provided for listing the attachments and innervation of muscles. Each exercise is followed by a section called **FOR REVIEW AND THOUGHT** in which the student is to actively review key items individually or with a partner. The overall intent is to thoroughly involve the learner in the material.

The modified outline format to this book is the key to its goals. Such a format allows an instructor to eliminate a particular section that his/her course may not deal with or to accentuate a section he/she considers more important than others. From the student's point of view this format allows nearly immediate access to facts without wading through voluminous textual material. It is the authors' hope that this approach will provide teacher and student with an enjoyable and challenging foray into the study of human anatomy.

The ideas and methods incorporated in this book incubated in the authors' minds for several years where they were kept warm by frequent discussion and criticism and the advice of colleagues. The authors would especially like to thank Dr. Robert Tallitsch, Augustance College, Rock Island, Illinois and Dr. Jerry A. Maynard, University of Iowa, Iowa City, Iowa for their willingness to read the draft manuscript and their helpful suggestions.

The manuscript was typed by Mrs. Sandra Swets, paste-up and cover design by David Carlson and photography by Jerry Mead. We thank them for their patience and understanding during the generation of the final manuscript.

Special thanks are due Mr. George Mundorff, Executive Editor, Lea and Febiger, who embraced this effort with enthusiasm and provided encouragement and guidance. We are also grateful to Dorothy DiRienzi, Copy Editor, and Tom Colaiezzi, Production Manager, Lea and Febiger for their assistance and to all at the Publisher who aided in the production of this book.

*Ann Arbor, Michigan*
*Fort Collins, Colorado*

ALAN TWIETMEYER
THOMAS MCCRACKEN

# CONTENTS

# TERMINOLOGY

## To The Student

The teaching and learning of anatomy is communicated through a language derived nearly exclusively from Latin and Greek. The following pages provide you with a listing of common root words, prefixes, and suffixes you will encounter in your studies. Each listing gives the Latin or Greek derivation and an example usage. Notice that each listing also has a blank line for you to become "actively involved" by adding another word or term as you learn it. This list is by no means complete so be prepared to add to it. Use the language of anatomy to help you learn (practice "Anglicizing" the Latin or Greek terms, example: biceps brachii = two headed muscle of the arm). Your success in learning anatomy will be closely linked to your success in using the language.

# COMMON ANATOMIC VOCABULARY

|  | Source | Example Terms |
|---|---|---|
| a- (an-) | G. without, not | anemia |
|  |  | _____ |
| ab- | L. from | abduct |
|  |  | _____ |
| acro- | G. extremity, tip | acromion process |
|  |  | _____ |
| ad- | L. to, toward | adduct |
|  |  | _____ |
| aden- | G. gland | adenoid |
|  |  | _____ |
| adipo- | L. fat | adipose |
|  |  | _____ |
| ambi- | L. both | ambidextrous |
|  |  | _____ |
| ante- | L. before, forward | anteversion |
|  |  | _____ |
| anti- | G. against | antiseptic |
|  |  | _____ |
| arthr- (arthro-) | G. a joint | arthritis |
|  |  | _____ |
| auto- | G. self | autonomic |
|  |  | _____ |
| bi- | L. two, double | bilateral |
|  |  | _____ |

| | Source | Example Terms |
|---|---|---|
| -blast | G. germ, bud | fibroblast |
| | | _____ |
| brachi- (brachion) | G. arm | brachial artery |
| | | _____ |
| brachium | L. arm | _____ |
| brevis | L. short | peroneus brevis |
| | | _____ |
| capit (caput) | L. head | semispinalis capitis |
| | | _____ |
| cervix | L. neck | cervix of uterus |
| | | _____ |
| chondro- | L. cartilage | chondrocyte |
| | | _____ |
| circum- | L. around, about | circumflex |
| | | _____ |
| -clast | G. to break | osteoclast |
| | | _____ |
| contra- | L. against, opposed | contraception |
| | | _____ |
| costa | L. rib | intercostal |
| | | _____ |
| crus | L. leg | talocrural joint |
| | | _____ |
| crux | L. cross | cruciate |
| | | _____ |

|  | Source | Example Terms |
|---|---|---|
| delta | G. triangle | deltoid |
| | | _____ |
| di- | G. double, two | diencephalon |
| | | _____ |
| dia- | G. through, completely | diagnosis |
| | | _____ |
| dis- | L. separation | dissect |
| | | _____ |
| ect- | G. outside | ectoderm |
| | | _____ |
| -ectomy | G. excision, removal | hysterectomy |
| | | _____ |
| end- (ent-) | G. within | endothelium |
| | | _____ |
| epi- | G. upon | epicondyle |
| | | _____ |
| ex- (exo) | G. & L. out | exocrine |
| | | _____ |
| extra- | L. beyond, outward | extracellular |
| | | _____ |
| gastr- (gastro-) | G. stomach | gastritis |
| | | _____ |
| hist- (histo-) | G. tissue | histology |
| | | _____ |

| | Source | Example Terms |
|---|---|---|
| hyal- (hyalo-) | G. glossy, clear | hyaline cartilage |
| | | _____ |
| hydro- | G. water | hydrocephalus |
| | | _____ |
| hyper- | G. above, over | hypertrophy |
| | | _____ |
| hypo- | G. under, less | hypobaric |
| | | _____ |
| im-, in- | L. intro | incision |
| | | _____ |
| im-, in- | L. negation, not | immature, involuntary |
| | | _____ |
| infra- | L. below | infraspinatus |
| | | _____ |
| inter- | L. between | intercondylar |
| | | _____ |
| intr- (intra-) | L. within | intravenous |
| | | _____ |
| linea | L. line | linea aspera |
| | | _____ |
| macro- | G. large | macrophage |
| | | _____ |
| medi- | G. middle | median |
| | | _____ |

|  | Source | Example Terms |
|---|---|---|
| meta- | G. changed, beyond | metatarsal |
|  |  | _____ |
| micro- | G. small | microbiology |
|  |  | _____ |
| myo- | G. muscle | myotome |
|  |  | _____ |
| nephr- | G. kidney | nephron |
|  |  | _____ |
| -oid | G. line, appearance, form | adenoid |
|  |  | _____ |
| para- | G. beside | paravertebral |
|  |  | _____ |
| peri- | G. around | perichondrium |
|  |  | _____ |
| -physis | G. to grow | pubic symphysis |
|  |  | _____ |
| post- | L. after, behind | postnatal |
|  |  | _____ |
| pre- | L. before, in front of | preganglionic |
|  |  | _____ |
| pro- | G. before, in front of | pronephros |
|  |  | _____ |
| ram- | L. branch | ramus |
|  |  | _____ |

|  | Source | Example Terms |
|---|---|---|
| re- | L. again, back | recurrent |
| rect- | L. straight | rectus femoris |
| ren- | L. kidney | renal |
| retro- | L. back, backward | retroperitoneal |
| sect | L. to cut | dissect |
| sub- | L. under | subdural |
| super- | L. over, excessive | superficial |
| supra- | L. above | supraorbital |
| sym-, syn- | G. together | symphysis<br>synthesis |
| teres | L. round | ligamentum teres |
| trans- | L. across, through, beyond | transfusion |

|  | Source | Example Terms |
|---|---|---|
| ultra- | L. beyond, excess | ultrastructure |
|  |  | _____ |
| vas | L. duct, vessel | vas deferens |
|  |  | _____ |
| vent- (ventr-) | L. belly | ventral |
|  |  | _____ |

**UNIT ONE:  UPPER LIMB**

**EXERCISE 1.  BONES OF THE UPPER LIMB**

The adult human skeleton is composed of 206 individual bones which, for classification purposes, may be grouped into axial and appendicular portions.  The axial skeleton includes the skull, vertebral column, sternum and ribs while the appendicular skeleton includes the bones of the limbs and their appropriate girdles.  The pectoral and pelvic girdles serve to join the upper and lower limbs, respectively, to the axial skeleton.

The skeleton serves five major purposes; hemopoiesis, mineral reservoir, support, protection, and movement.  Obviously not all bones share in these purposes equally and this fact plus their location in the body determine their shape.  A common classification of bones by shape follows:

**Long** - consist of a body (shaft) and two ends; found in the limbs

**Short** - do not have a long axis; found in the wrist and ankle

**Flat** - ribs; sternum; bones of cranium

**Irregular** - vertebrae; scapula; pelvis; facial bones

As you study bones get in the habit of mentally classifying them by shape, location, and function.  Bones possess certain landmarks caused by muscle attachments, passage of blood vessels or nerves, association with tendons, union with another bone, etc..  Given on page 2 is a list of terms used to describe these landmarks.  As you encounter each term fill in the definition and an example of a bone possessing such a landmark.

| Term | Definition | Example |
|------|-----------|---------|
| spine | an abrupt or pointed projection | scapular spine |
| process | | |
| tubercle | | |
| tuberosity | | |
| fossa | | |
| foramen | | |
| sulcus | | |
| trochanter | | |
| line | | |
| crest | | |
| condyle | | |
| epicondyle | | |

Now, find the following on the skeletal materials provided and label the figures in this exercise properly.

I. **Scapula (Figures 1.1 and 1.2)**

    A. **Superior border**

    B. **Superior angle**

    C. **Vertebral border**

    D. **Axillary border**

    E. **Inferior angle**

    F. **Scapular spine**

    G. **Acromion process**

    H. **Coracoid process**

    I. **Supraspinous fossa**

    J. **Infraspinous fossa**

    K. **Subscapular fossa**

    L. **Glenoid fossa**

    M. **Supraglenoid tubercle**

    N. **Infraglenoid tubercle**

    O. **Scapular (Suprascapular) notch**

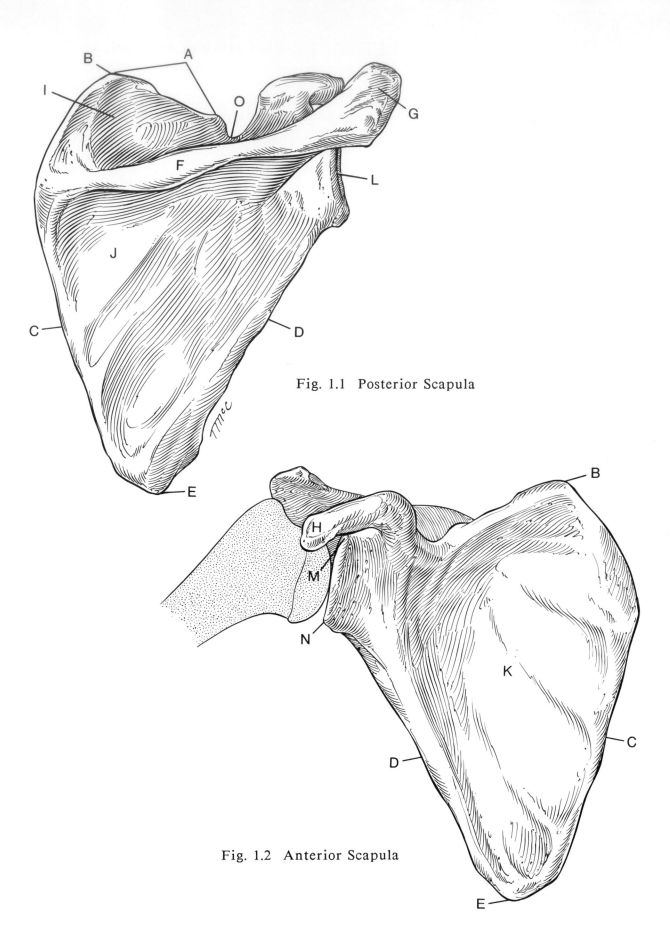

Fig. 1.1  Posterior Scapula

Fig. 1.2  Anterior Scapula

4

## II. Clavicle (Figure 1.3)

A. **Sternal end**

B. **Acromial end**

C. **Conoid tubercle**

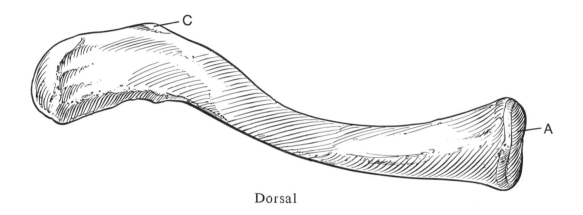

Dorsal

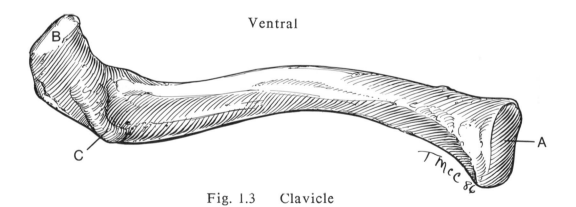

Ventral

Fig. 1.3    Clavicle

III. Humerus, Radius, Ulna (Figures 1.4 and 1.5)

Humerus

A. Head

B. Anatomical neck

C. Surgical neck

D. Greater and lesser tubercles

E. Intertubercular (Bicipital) groove

F. Deltoid tuberosity

G. Body - with radial groove

H. Medial and lateral epicondyles and supracondylar ridges

I. Condyle

    1. Capitulum

    2. Trochlea

J. Coronoid fossa

K. Radial fossa

L. Olecranon fossa

Radius

M. Head

N. Neck

O. Radial tuberosity

P. Body

Q. Carpal articular surface

R. Ulnar notch

S. Styloid process

Ulna

T. Olecranon process

U. Coronoid process

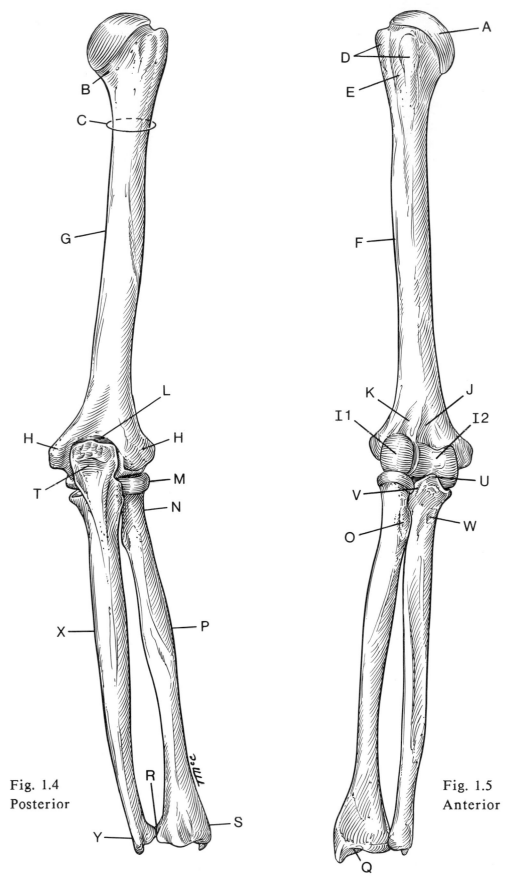

Fig. 1.4
Posterior

Fig. 1.5
Anterior

Humerus; Radius; Ulna

V.    **Radial notch**

W.    **Ulnar tuberosity**

X.    **Body**

Y.    **Head** - with styloid process

IV.  **Carpal (wrist) Bones (Figures 1.6 and 1.7)**

**Proximal Row**

A.    **Scaphoid (navicular)**

B.    **Lunate**

C.    **Triquetral (triquetrum)**

D.    **Pisiform**

**Distal Row**

E.    **Trapezium**

F.    **Trapezoid**

G.    **Capitate**

H.    **Hamate**

V.  **Metacarpals (Figures 1.6 and 1.7)**

Numbered 1-5 from radial side to ulnar side. Each has a base (proximal), body, and head (distal).

VI.  **Phalanges (Figures 1.6 and 1.7)**

Numbered as are the metacarapals. Digit one (1) has only two phalanges (proximal and distal) while the other four digits (2-5) have proximal, middle, and distal phalanges.

## FOR REVIEW AND THOUGHT

Study the bones involved in the joints of the upper limb. What bones articulate at the shoulder, elbow, wrist, and metacarpal-phalangeal joint of the thumb? What movements are allowed at each of these joints? Which joints of the upper limb are designed for mobility and which for stability? Which joint of the upper limb is most often injured?

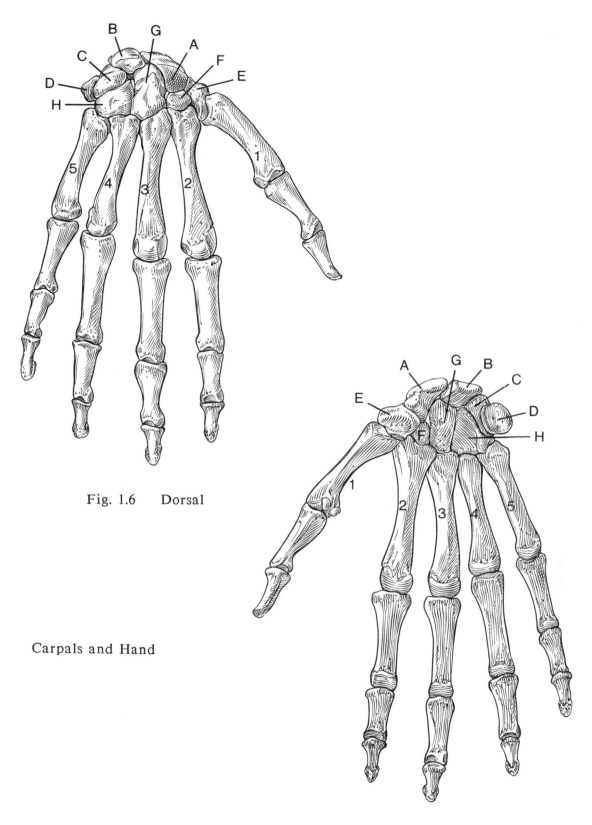

Fig. 1.6    Dorsal

Carpals and Hand

Fig. 1.7    Palmar

9

# EXERCISE 2. MUSCLES OF THE PECTORAL GIRDLE AND SHOULDER

For our purposes the muscles of the pectoral girdle are considered to be any that serve to position or stabilize the clavicle and/or scapula. These muscles may be located on the anterior thoracic wall or superficially on the back.

Muscles are often described as having an origin and an insertion. In this concept the origin is defined as the more proximal (or stable) attachment and the insertion as the more distal or peripheral attachment (which is usually more moveable). Which attachment is the more moveable is often dependent upon factors such as gravity and weight bearing, thus causing confusion regarding origin and insertion. For this reason the authors prefer to describe attachments as simply proximal and distal.

Before beginning this exercise review the terminology from **Exercise 1** relating to the scapula, clavicle, and humerus.

## I. Anterior Muscles (Figures 2.1 and 2.2)

### A.   Pectoralis major (*                    )

This large and powerful muscle has an extensive proximal attachment and a more limited distal attachment, which allows a greater range of possible actions of this muscle; observe these attachments and describe them below.

    PA -


    DA -


As inferred above this muscle is capable of producing several movements. Are these movements related to specific portions of the muscle?

### B.   Pectoralis minor (                    )

This muscle is located deep to the pectoralis major and serves as the gateway to the axilla; it is an important landmark structure.

    PA -


    DA -

*This space provided for writing the innervation of the muscle. See p. 27.

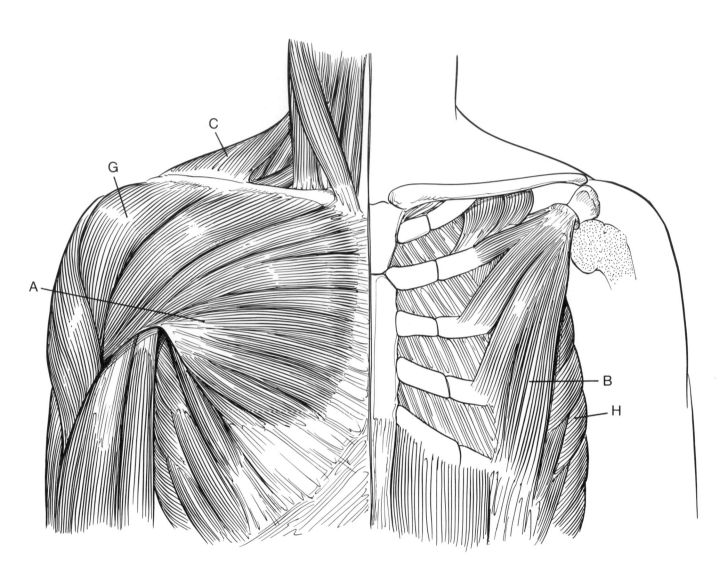

Fig. 2.1  Muscles, Anterior Thorax and Shoulder

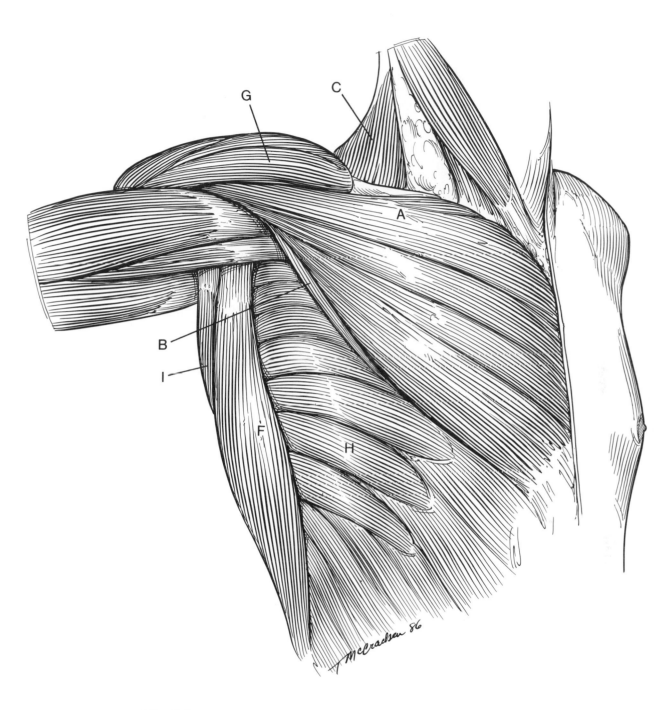

Fig. 2.2    Muscles, Lateral Thorax and Shoulder

13

## II. Posterior Muscles (Figures 2.2 and 2.3)

### C. Trapezius (                                    )

The trapezius is superficially situated on the posterior neck and thorax. Like the pectoralis major it has a vast proximal attachment and a more limited distal attachment. When the two trapezius muscles are viewed together they appear as a trapezoid, thus their name. Each trapezius is often described as having superior, middle, and inferior portions based upon different distal attachments. Study the trapezius muscle and list its attachments below.

PA -

DA -

Deep to the trapezius are several other important muscles.

### D. Levator scapulae (                                    )

This muscle takes its proximal attachment off the transverse processes of the cervical vertebrae. What is the distal attachment of this muscle?

DA -

### E. Rhomboids (major and minor)  (                                    )

These two muscles (each shaped like a rhombus but differing in size) have their distal attachment along the medial (vertebral) border of the scapula. Describe below the specifics of these distal attachments as well as proximal attachments.

PA -

DA -

### F. Latissimus dorsi (                                    )

This powerful muscle is also located on the back but is a muscle of the upper limb. The proximal attachment of this muscle passes inferiorly from approximately the T6 vertebra to the sacrum. Additionally a portion of this muscle often has a proximal attachment on the inferior angle of the scapula. What is the distal attachment of the latissimus dorsi?

DA -

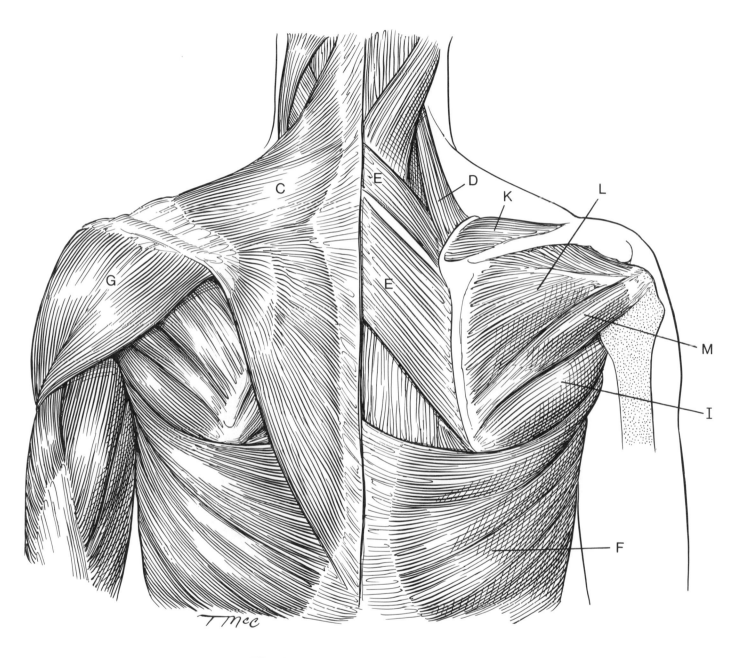

Fig. 2.3    Muscles, Posterior
Thorax and Shoulder

15

From what you have learned regarding the pectoralis major and trapezius what does such an arrangement of attachments tell you about the latissimus dorsi?

G.  **Deltoid** (                                    )

The triangularly shaped deltoid gives the rounded contour to the shoulder; it is often described as having anterior, middle, and posterior portions based upon differing proximal attachments.  List the proximal attachment of each portion below and the distal attachment of the entire muscle.

PA -

DA -

Given these attachments, can you perceive the different movements that would be brought about by each portion?

H.  **Serratus anterior** (                                    )

This muscle is difficult to visualize and appreciate because its distal attachment is on the deep surface of the medial border of the scapula; you will find its serrated proximal attachment on the lateral side of the thorax from ribs 2-8.

I.  **Teres major** (                                    )

The teres major lies deep to the latissimus dorsi and is partially obscured by it.  Find the proximal attachment on the inferior aspect of the axillary border of the scapula and trace the muscle to its distal attachment.  Write its distal attachment below.

DA -

The final muscles to be discussed in this exercise are those of the rotator cuff.  This term is partially a misnomer; the four muscles involved do indeed form a cuff over the superior and posterior aspects of the humeral head, but only three of the muscles produce rotation of the humerus.

J.  **Subscapularis** (                                    )

Like the serratus anterior, this muscle is difficult to visualize.  Its proximal attachment is off the subscapular fossa, which is on the anterior (deep, costal) surface of the scapula.  The distal attachment is on an important bony landmark of the humerus.  Write the distal attachment below.

DA -

**K.** **Supraspinatus (**                      **)**

This is the one muscle that is not a rotator of the humerus. Given its name what would you propose as its proximal attachment? What is its distal attachment? List them below.

PA -

DA -

If this muscle is not a rotator of the humerus, what is its function? Use the attachments of the muscle to help you determine this.

**L.** **Infraspinatus (**                   **)**

Like the supraspinatus the name of this muscle tells you its proximal attachment. List the attachments below.

PA -

DA -

**M.** **Teres minor (**                    **)**

The distal attachment of this muscle is just inferior to that of the infraspinatus. What is its proximal attachment?

PA -

DA -

As you have seen by now the three muscles you have just found all have their distal attachment on the greater tubercle of the humerus from superior to inferior. This can be remembered by the word SIT, standing for supraspinatus, infraspinatus, and teres minor. The remaining muscle of the rotator cuff, the subscapularis, has its distal attachment on the lesser tubercle. Note, the teres major is a rotator of the humerus but is not a member of the rotator cuff.

## FOR REVIEW AND THOUGHT

You have had an introduction to the following muscles:

**Pectoralis major**

**Pectoralis minor**

**Trapezius (3 portions)**

**Deltoid (3 portions)**

**Rhomboids (major and minor)**

**Supraspinatus**

**Infraspinatus**

**Teres minor**

**Teres major**

**Latissimus dorsi**

**Levator scapulae**

**Serratus anterior**

**Subscapularis**

Each of these muscles has all or part of one of its attachments on the pectoral girdle (scapula and clavicle). From this information decide which of these muscles function in positioning the girdle and which in positioning the humerus. Write the answers next to each muscle. Additionally, by studying the attachments, begin to develop a picture of what movements each of these muscles might produce and, conversely, what movements they might oppose. Write these movements next to each muscle and discuss them with your laboratory/study partners.

### <u>NOTES</u>

# EXERCISE 3. AXILLARY REGION; ARM

The axillary region is commonly known as the armpit. The axilla is a cone-shaped area through which the blood vessels and nerves to the upper limb pass, accompanied by a number of lymph nodes and channels. The apex of this cone is immediately superior to the first rib. The boundaries of the axilla are the pectoralis minor and major anteriorly; the subscapularis, teres major, and latissimus dorsi posteriorly; the thoracic wall with overlying serratus anterior medially; and the humerus laterally. Prior to beginning this exercise review the location, attachments, and functions of the muscles just mentioned.

In dissections, to see clearly the contents of the axilla two things must be done: first the gateway to the axilla (pectoralis minor) must be moved out of the way, and second the axillary sheath, a layer of loose connective tissue enveloping the nerves and vessels, must be removed. When this has been done the contents of the axilla are more apparent. These contents are: brachial plexus, axillary artery and vein, lymph nodes, and some fat. The lymph nodes of the region are important in the metastasis (spreading; moving) of carcinoma (cancer) of the breast.

We will begin the study of this region with perhaps the most complicated, yet interesting, group of structures: the brachial plexus. The brachial plexus is composed of the neural elements that combine and branch to form the nerve supply to the upper limb. For the moment let us learn the rudiments of the plexus in outline format.

I. **Brachial Plexus (Figure 3.1)**

    A.   **Origin** - ventral primary rami of cervical nerves 5-8 and thoracic nerve 1 (C5-T1)

    B.   **ROOTS - join to form TRUNKS**

        1.   Superior trunk - C5,6

        2.   Middle trunk   - C7

        3.   Inferior trunk - C8,T1

    C.   **TRUNKS - split to form DIVISIONS**

        4.   Anterior divisions - nerves from these are destined to supply anterior (flexor) muscles

        5.   Posterior divisions - nerves from these are destined to supply posterior (extensor) muscles

    D.   **DIVISIONS - join to form CORDS**

        6.   Lateral cord - formed by anterior divisions of the superior and middle trunks

        7.   Medial cord - formed by the anterior division of the inferior trunk

        8.   Posterior cord - formed by the posterior divisions of all three trunks

E. **CORDS give off TERMINAL BRANCHES**

**from the lateral cord**

9. Musculocutaneous nerve - motor to anterior arm muscles

10a. 1/2 of the median nerve

**from the medial cord**

10b. 1/2 of the median nerve - the median nerve is motor to most of the anterior forearm muscles; thenar muscles; and lateral two lumbricals

11. Ulnar nerve - motor to 1 1/2 muscles of the anterior forearm; intrinsic muscles of the hand; and medial two lumbricals

**from the posterior cord**

12. Axillary nerve - motor to the deltoid and teres minor

13. Radial nerve - motor to the posterior muscles of the arm and forearm

F. **COLLATERAL BRANCHES** - from **ROOTS, TRUNKS,** and **CORDS,** but not from **DIVISIONS**

**from roots**

14. Dorsal scapular nerve - from C5; motor to the rhomboids and levator scapula

15. Long thoracic nerve - from C5-C7; motor to the serratus anterior

**from trunks**

16. Suprascapular nerve - from the superior trunk; motor to the supraspinatus and infraspinatus

17. Nerve to the subclavius - from the superior trunk; motor to the subclavius

**from the lateral cord**

18. Lateral pectoral nerve - motor to the pectoralis major

**from the medial cord**

19. Medial pectoral nerve - motor to the pectoralis major and minor

20. Medial brachial cutaneous - sensory to the medial surface of the arm

21. Medial antebrachial cutaneous - sensory to the medial surface of the forearm

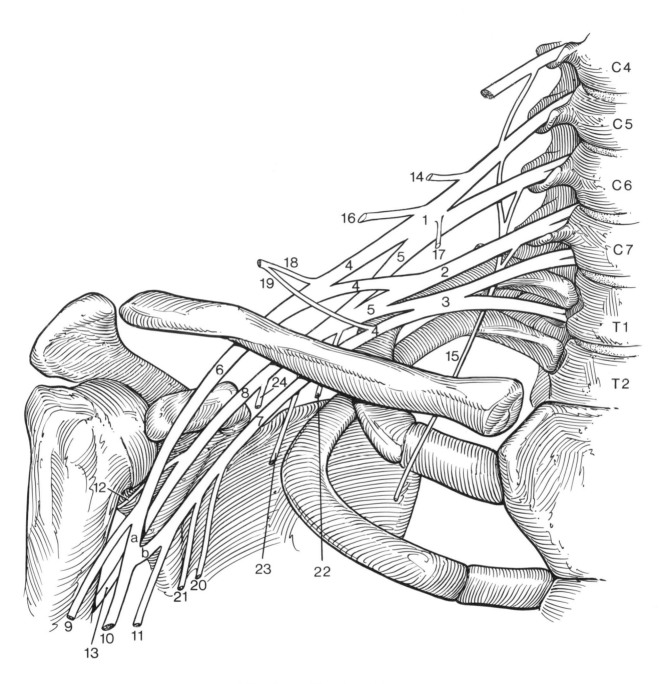

Fig. 3.1    Brachial Plexus

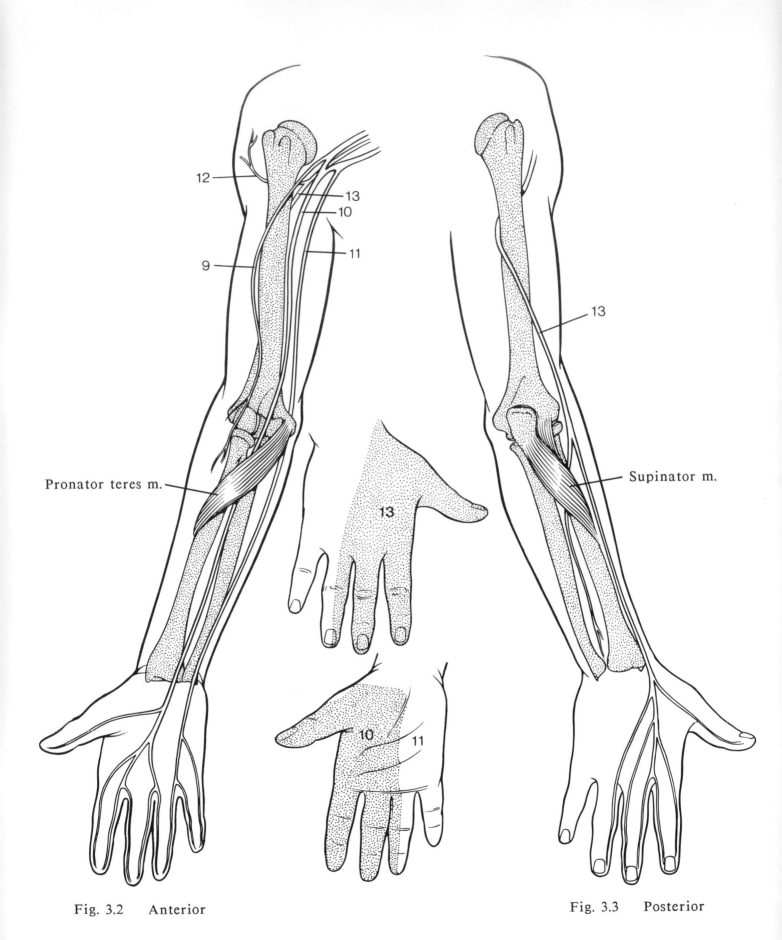

Pronator teres m.

Supinator m.

12

13
10
11

9

13

13

10    11

Fig. 3.2    Anterior

Fig. 3.3    Posterior

Nerve Course and Distribution

22.    Upper subscapular nerve - motor to the subscapularis

23.    Thoracodorsal nerve - motor to the latissimus dorsi

24.    Lower subscapular nerve - motor to the subscapularis and teres major

As you study the muscles of the upper limb continue to think of the brachial plexus in outline form; it will aid you in learning the nerve supply of the muscles. Refer to the diagram of the brachial plexus (Figure 3.1) and label the structures. Whenever studying the plexus orient yourself by finding the "M" made by the musculocutaneous, median, and ulnar nerves (from lateral to medial). From this "M" you can work proximally to find the cords and distally to trace these three nerves. Use Figures 3.2 and 3.3 to label and study the distribution of the five terminal branches of the brachial plexus.

## II.  Vascular Structures (Figures 3.4 and 3.5)

The vascular structures for the upper limb also pass through the axilla: axillary artery and vein. The axillary artery (Figure 3.4), a continuation of the subclavian artery as it passes over the first rib, is positioned between the cords of the brachial plexus, and the cords are named for their positions relative to this artery.

For conceptual and organizational purposes the axillary artery is described in three parts with each part having specific branches arising from it. Interestingly, and conveniently for learning, the first part has one branch, the second part two branches, and the third part three branches. Below is a table listing the boundaries of the three parts of the axillary artery. Write in the branches from each part as you learn them. (A complete outline of the arterial and venous structures of the upper limb is presented on pages 42-44).

**Part One**
**Boundaries**                                      **Branches**

from the lateral surface
of the first rib to the
superior surface of the
pectoralis minor

**Part Two**
**Boundaries**                                      **Branches**

posterior to the
pectoralis minor

**Part Three**
**Boundaries**                                      **Branches**

from the inferior border
of the pectoralis minor
to the inferior border
of the teres major

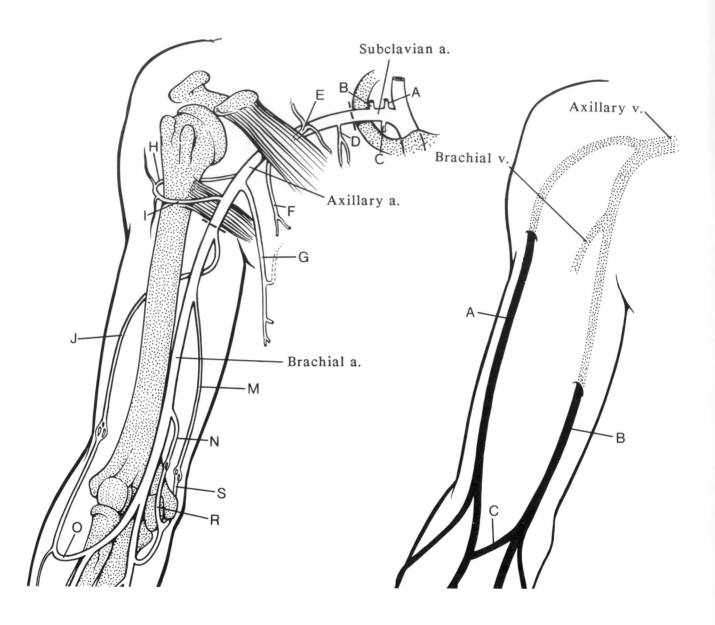

Subclavian a.

E B A

H

I

F

Axillary a.

G

J

Brachial a.

M

N

S

R

O

Axillary v.

Brachial v.

A

B

C

Fig. 3.4    Arterial Supply,
Arm

Fig. 3.5    Superficial Venous Drainage,
Arm

24

As the axillary artery crosses the inferior border of the teres major it enters the arm and is then called the brachial artery. (A complete outline of the arterial and venous structures of the upper limb is presented on pages 42-44.)

The axillary vein (Figure 3.5) receives venous drainage from the upper limb. This drainage is from both superficial (basilic and cephalic) and deep (brachial) veins. The axillary vein is usually considered to be a continuation of the basilic vein which is joined by the brachial vein at about the same point. The cephalic vein empties into the axillary vein, which becomes the subclavian vein as it crosses the first rib. (A complete outline of the arterial and venous structures of the upper limb is presented on pages 42-44).

## III. Muscles of the Arm (Figures 3.6 and 3.7)

The arm is the region between the shoulder and elbow. The muscles of the arm function at either/both the shoulder and/or elbow.

### A. Triceps brachii (                          )

This three headed muscle is found on the posterior surface of the arm. Only one of its three heads has a proximal attachment on the scapula. Which one? _____ The other two heads have their proximal attachments on the shaft of the humerus.

1. Long head

2. Medial head

3. Lateral head

What is the distal attachment of the triceps brachii as a whole? _____ Given this, what is the function of the triceps brachii? _____

### B. Biceps brachii (                          )

The biceps brachii is located superficially and anteriorly in the arm. The heads have separate proximal attachments and a common distal attachment; list them below.

4. Long head - PA -

5. Short head - PA -

DA -

At what joints does the biceps brachii act and what movements does it produce? _____

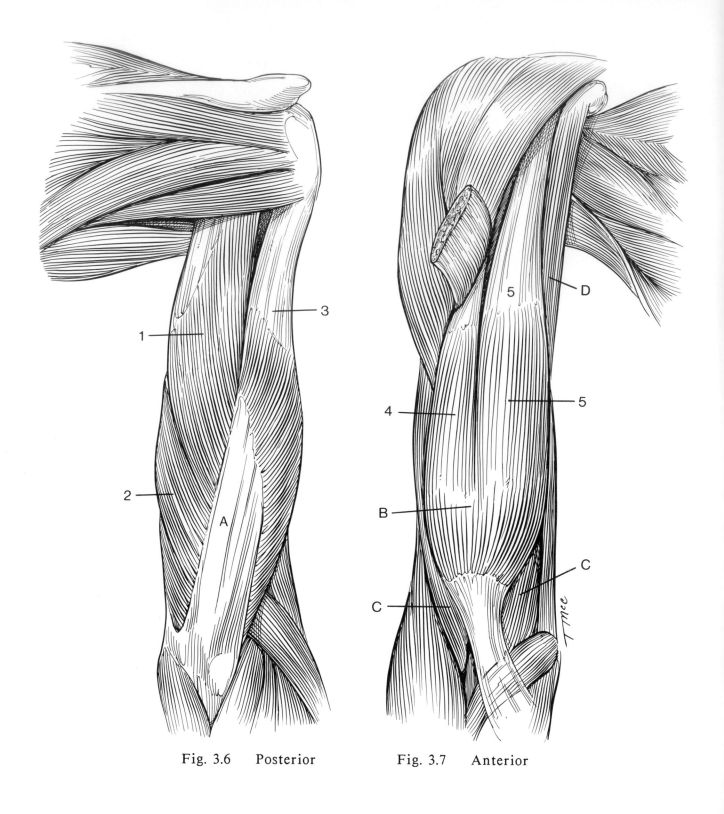

Fig. 3.6   Posterior          Fig. 3.7   Anterior

Muscles, Deep Shoulder and Arm

C.  **Brachialis**  (                                        )

This muscle is found deep to the biceps brachii and is known as the "true flexor of the forearm." From this description alone what would you deduce as the proximal and distal attachments?

PA -


DA -

D.  **Coracobrachialis**  (                             )

This is the smallest muscle of the arm. Use the name of the muscle to learn the proximal and distal attachments and list them below.

PA -


DA -


## FOR REVIEW AND THOUGHT

You have now studied a key and complex region of the upper limb. In order to reinforce your learning return to sections **A**, **B**, **C**, and **D** above and in the spaces provided write the nerve supply to each muscle and the cord from which the nerve arises. Then do the same for the following muscles:

**Deltoid**            (                                        )

**Teres minor**        (                                        )

**Teres major**        (                                        )

**Subscapularis**      (                                        )

**Latissimus dorsi**   (                                        )

Similarly return to the muscles you learned in **Exercise 2** and write their innervation and the portion of the brachial plexus from which each nerve arises. You will notice that the trapezius is not innervated by a branch from any portion of the brachial plexus. The nerve supply to the trapezius is from the XI cranial nerve, Spinal Accessory.

Discuss with your laboratory or study partners the relationship of nerve injury to functional loss in the region. Pose your questions this way: If the lateral cord of the brachial plexus was damaged in the axilla, what functional loss might be shown at the shoulder joint? Develop this method of question and answer now as it will serve you well as we proceed distally in the limb.

# EXERCISE 4. FOREARM, WRIST AND HAND

Before beginning this exercise review the bones of the forearm and hand (**Exercise 1**). Your understanding of the muscles of this region, and their actions, will be facilitated by a knowledge of these bones. Of special importance are the following:

The radius rotates about the longitudinal axis of the ulna in supination-pronation; the hand is carried along by the radius.

The main articulation of the forearm to the wrist is that between the radius and scaphoid.

The carpal-metacarpal joint of the thumb occurs between the trapezium and first metacarpal. This is the most moveable of all carpal-metacarpal joints! Why? What is the significance of this mobility?

For our purposes extrinsic and intrinsic muscles of the hand will be defined thusly:

Extrinsic - those muscles with their proximal attachment on the arm or forearm and distal attachment on the carpals, metacarpals, or phalanges

Intrinsic - those muscles with both proximal and distal attachments on carpals, metacarpals, and phalanges

## I. Flexor Aspect of the Forearm (Figures 4.1 and 4.2)

The muscles of the flexor forearm are neatly arranged in four layers. In general, as you proceed from superficial to deep, the muscles of each layer act more distally in the limb; this is not so for the deepest (fourth) layer. The brackets are provided for you to note the innervation of each muscle.

A. **Superficial group (first layer)** - The four muscles of the superficial group all have complete or partial proximal attachment off the medial epicondyle of the humerus. Study these muscles and list the distal attachments of each.

1. Pronator teres ( )

   DA -

2. Flexor carpi radialis ( )

   DA -

3. Palmaris longus ( )

   DA -

4. Flexor carpi ulnaris ( )

   DA -

Because of differing distal attachments these muscles have differing functions, but with a similar proximal attachment they are all capable, to varying degrees,

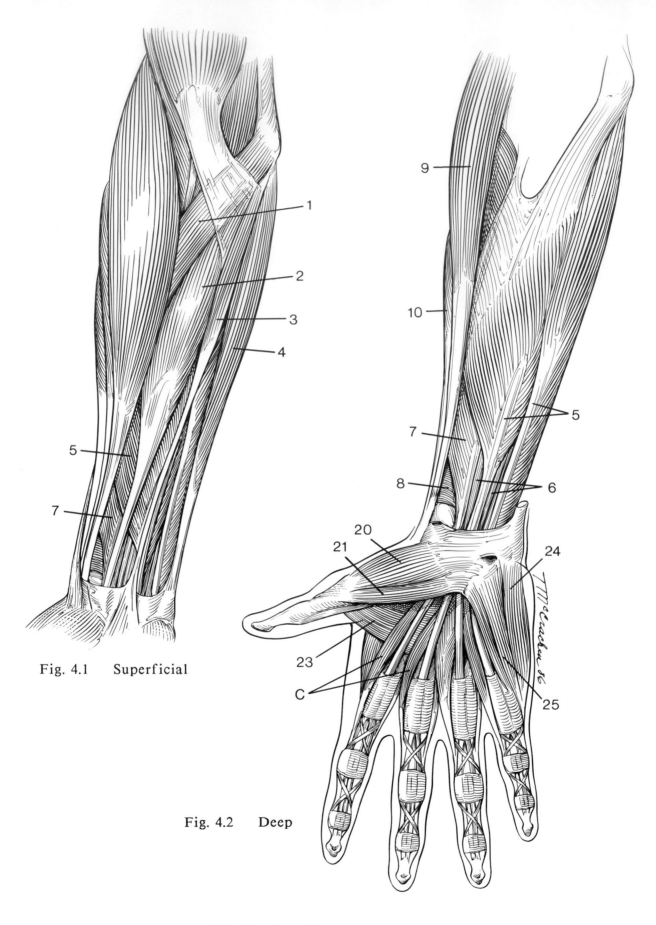

Fig. 4.1    Superficial

Fig. 4.2    Deep

Muscles, Anterior Forearm and Hand

30

of a particular function at the elbow. What is that function? _____
_____

B. **Second layer** - Only one muscle is found in the second layer: the flexor digitorum superficialis (sublimis). The former is probably the more common usage, but the latter may aid you in learning the function of this muscle in that it has a more sublime action on the phalanges. The belly of this muscle takes proximal attachment partly off the medial epicondyle of the humerus and partly off the radius and ulna. The muscle splits into four tendons which pass into the hand to attach where distally?

    5.    Flexor digitorum superficialis (                       )

       DA -

C. **Third layer** - Two muscles occupy this layer: the flexor digitorum profundus (the profound flexor of the digits) and the flexor pollicis longus. In addition the median and ulnar nerves are found in association with these muscles. The median nerve is found between these muscles, and the ulnar nerve on the medial side of the flexor digitorum profundus, accompanied closely by the ulnar artery. The flexor digitorum profundus takes its proximal attachment from the ulna and interosseus membrane while the flexor pollicis longus is attached to the radius. Write the distal attachments of these muscles below.

    6.    Flexor digitorum profundus (             )

       DA -

    7.    Flexor pollicis longus (             )

       DA -

D. **Fourth layer** - As with the second layer only one muscle is found in the fourth layer, the pronator quadratus. The name of this muscle tells you both its function and its shape. List below the attachments of this muscle.

    8.    Pronator quadratus (             )

       PA -

       DA -

II. **Extensor Aspect of the Forearm (Figures 4.2 and 4.3)**

The muscles of the extensor forearm are also arranged in layers, although this arrangement is complicated somewhat by a group of "outcropping muscles" that act on the thumb.

A. **Superficial group (first layer)** - All of these muscles have complete or partial attachment off the lateral epicondyle of the humerus. Again, as with the flexor forearm, the muscles lying deeper have their action on more distal portions of the limb.

9. Brachioradialis ( )

PA -

DA -

Because of these attachments this muscle is a flexor at the elbow even though it is described with the extensor muscles and is innervated by the nerve to the extensors. In what position of the forearm is it most effective? _____
Be sure you understand these concepts before you proceed!

10. Extensor carpi radialis longus ( )

PA -

DA -

11. Extensor carpi radialis brevis ( )

PA -

DA -

12. Extensor digitorum communis ( )

This muscle splits into four tendons, prominently visible on the dorsum of the hand, which attach via an intricate arrangement known as the extensor expansion. Describe the proximal and distal attachments of this muscle below. Note also the intertendinous connections limiting independent extension of the fingers.

PA -

DA -

13. Extensor carpi ulnaris ( )

PA -

DA -

14. Extensor digiti minimi ( )

The tendon of this muscle may arise from the belly of the extensor digitorum communis.

PA -

DA -

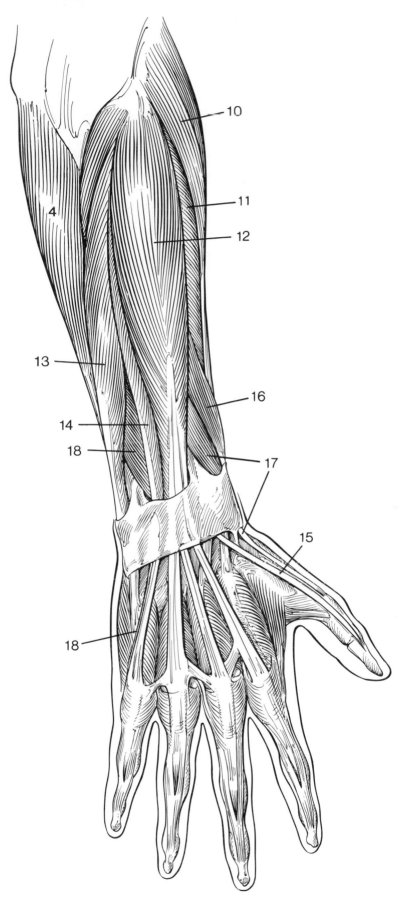

Fig. 4.3    Muscles, Superficial Posterior
Forearm and Hand

33

B.  **Second layer** - This layer includes the "outcropping muscles," the proper extensor of the index finger, and the supinator. The "outcropping muscles" form a bulge on the posterolateral surface of the inferior forearm. These muscles have their proximal attachments on the radius and interosseous membrane and distal attachments, via prominent tendons, onto the thumb. These tendons form the boundaries of an area at the base of the thumb called the "anatomical snuff box." Gentlemen of earlier eras put their snuff in this depression. Of more significance to the present discussion is the fact the radial artery passes through the snuffbox and the pulse can be felt here by pressing the artery against the deeper lying trapezium and scaphoid.

15. Extensor pollicis longus (                                )

The posterior boundary of the snuffbox is formed by its tendon, which passes to the thumb for distal attachment on the

_____.

16. Abductor pollicis longus (                        )

Along with the tendon of the extensor pollicis brevis this muscle forms the anterior boundary of the snuffbox. Write the distal attachment below.

DA -

17. Extensor pollicis brevis (                        )

DA -

18. Extensor indicis proprius (                        )

As noted above the extensor digitorum communis is characterized by several intertendinous connections, limiting independent extension of the involved digits. The index finger (second digit) is provided with a second extensor, the "proper extensor of the index finger." Thus the second digit is usually the only one capable of independent extension. Write in the attachments of this muscle below.

PA -

DA -

19. Supinator (                        )

This is the deepest muscle of the posterior forearm. The radial nerve usually pierces the muscle as it enters the forearm (Figure 3.3). The attachments of this muscle are:

PA -

DA -

You have now studied four muscles with major functions in either pronation or supination.  List those muscles!

_____

_____

_____

_____

What do all these muscles have in common regarding their distal attachments?

C.    <u>Radial nerve and artery</u> - Unlike the ulnar nerve and artery the radial nerve and artery do not travel together in the forearm.  The nerve is seen to emerge from the posterior surface of the humerus between the brachioradialis and brachialis and to pierce the supinator before giving muscular branches to the extensor muscles.  One major branch, the posterior interosseous, continues to provide motor supply as it proceeds distally to end as a sensory supply to a small area on the dorsum of the hand.  The radial artery branches from the brachial artery distal to the elbow and passes deep in the extensor compartment. It becomes superficial in the snuffbox and continues into the hand, where it contributes to the superficial and deep palmar arches (see **Circulatory System Outline, Upper Limb,** pp. 42-44).

## III. Hand (Figures 4.2 - 4.6)

The intrinsic muscles of the hand may be arranged in four groups:  thenar (thumb), hypothenar (little finger), lumbricals, and interossei.  The need to learn specific attachments of each of these muscles will be determined by professional and educational objectives.  Most important, in the authors' view,  is to understand functions and the implications of nerve damage on these functions.

A.    **Thenar muscles (Figure 4.2)** - Four intrinsic muscles act to position the thumb. Three of these muscles are found in the thenar eminence, the raised pad at the base of the thumb.  Notice that the palmar surface of the thumb is turned 90 degrees to those of the other digits.  Thus the various movements of the thumb occur in a different plane than similar movements of the other digits. To verify this flex digits 2-5 then flex the thumb; similarly for extension, abduction, and adduction.  The thumb is capable of an important additional movement: opposition.  Opposition of the thumb brings the palmar surface in contact with the palmar surfaces of the other digits.

20.   Abductor pollicis brevis

21.   Flexor pollicis brevis

These two muscles are the most superficial in the thenar eminence. Their distal attachments are on the appropriate surface of the proximal phalanx to produce the movement described by their name.

22.   Opponens pollicis

This muscle is found immediately deep to the abductor and flexor. These three muscles are innervated by what nerve? _____

_____

23.   Adductor pollicis

The adductor pollicis is a thenar muscle but is not found in the thenar eminence. It is found on the palmar side of the gap between the first and second metacarpals. As with all the thenar muscles its function is obvious by its name. What is the nerve supply of this muscle? _____

_____

B.   **Hypothenar muscles (Figure 4.2)** - The hypothenar eminence, at the base of the little finger, contains three muscles similar in function to those of the thenar eminence. The fifth digit is capable of limited opposition. As with the thenar muscles, the abductor and flexor are superficial and the opponens deep.

24.   Abductor digiti minimi (                              )

25.   Flexor digiti minimi (                              )

26.   Opponens digiti minimi (                              )

Write the nerve supply of these muscles in the space provided. Why is it different than that of the thenar muscles?

C.   **Lumbricals (Figures 4.2 and 4.6)** - The four lumbrical muscles are unique in attachments and in function. Up to this point you have studied extrinsic muscles of the hand, which either flex or extend at one or more joints. The intrinsic muscles you have just learned also produce one specific movement. The lumbricals are capable of producing flexion and extension at different joints at the same time. The four lumbricals take their proximal attachment off the radial side of what tendons? _____

From this attachment these small "worm-like" muscles pass anterior to the transverse axis of the metacarpophalangeal joint to reach their distal attachment on the _____ and the _____
_____. Thus these muscles are capable of producing flexion at the _____ and extension at the _____
_____ joints.

This capability is essential in allowing the hand to function in the variety of intricate activities it is involved in. The four lumbricals are innervated in accordance with the muscle from whose tendons they take attachment, the flexor digitorum profundus. Therefore the lateral two lumbricals are supplied by the _____ nerve and the medial two by the _____ _____ nerve.

D.  **Interossei (Figures 4.4 - 4.6)** - Seven interossei are usually described: three palmar and four dorsal. These muscles function primarily in abduction and adduction of the fingers, movements that are defined about a longitudinal line through the third finger. The interossei take proximal attachment off the metacarpals and attach distally to the appropriate side of a proximal phalanx to produce either abduction or adduction. The four dorsal interossei are abductors, a fact that can be remembered by the acronym DAB. Given their function, and the definition of abduction and adduction described above, to what sides of which proximal phalanges will these muscles attach? Remember, the thumb and little finger have their own named abductors.

The palmar interossei are adductors (acronym PAD). The thumb has its own named adductor. To what surfaces of which phalanges will these muscles attach?

In addition to these functions the interossei also assist the lumbricals because they pass anterior to the transverse axis of the metacarpophalangeal joint and attach distally in part into the extensor hood. What is the innervation of the interossei?

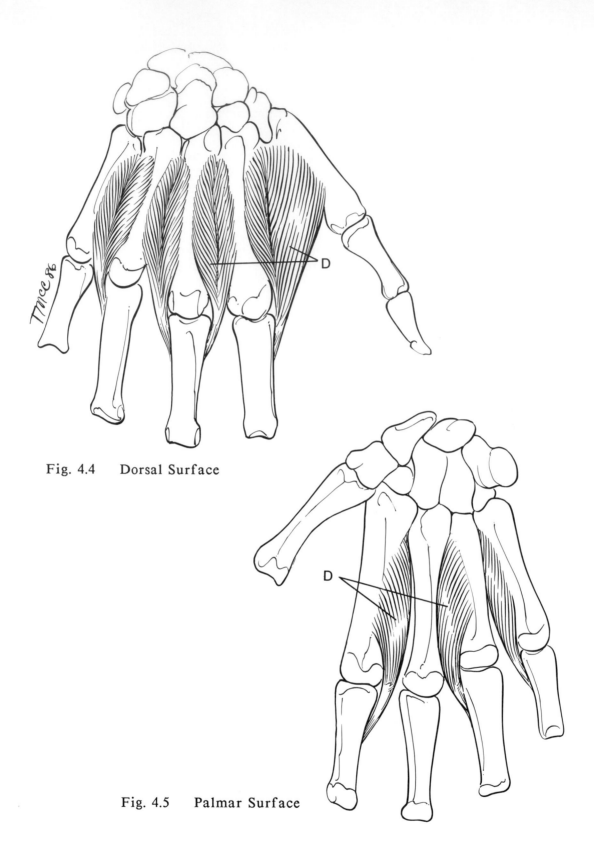

Fig. 4.4    Dorsal Surface

Fig. 4.5    Palmar Surface

Deep Muscles of the Hand

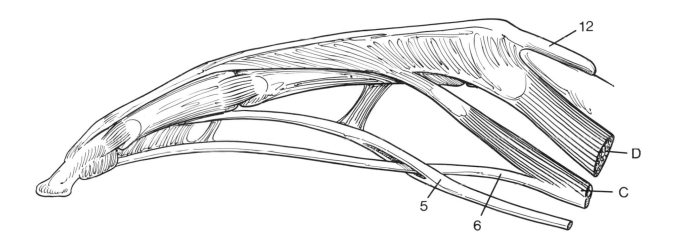

Fig. 4.6   Tendons of Finger

The numbers indicate tendons of muscles described
and shown previously (see pp. 29-31)

## FOR REVIEW AND THOUGHT

You have completed the study of the upper limb. While these exercises, by necessity, dealt with specific regions of the upper limb, it is important that you conceive of the upper limb as a functional unit and be able to trace certain structures along their course in the limb. Given below are some suggested subjects for discussion, questioning, and answering.

A. Which muscles of the upper limb are multiple joint muscles? What joints do they cross and what is their function at these joints?

B. What muscles function in various positions of the hand? In answering this question use your hand in various situations: hold a ball, grip a pencil, hold a hand of cards, etc.

C. Trace the following structures throughout their course in the limb. Describe their functional significance and important landmarks that might be used to locate them (use Figures 3.2 through 3.5 and 4.7 and 4.8 and label Figure 4.9).

1. Superficial veins (cephalic, basilic, median cubital)

2. Deep veins (brachial, axillary)

3. Arterial supply from the first rib to the hand

4. Axillary nerve

5. Radial nerve

6. Musculocutaneous nerve

7. Median nerve

8. Ulnar nerve

D. Study and label Figure 4.6 to assist you in understanding the involvement of the lumbricals and interossei in metacarpophalangeal flexion with concomitant interphalangeal extension.

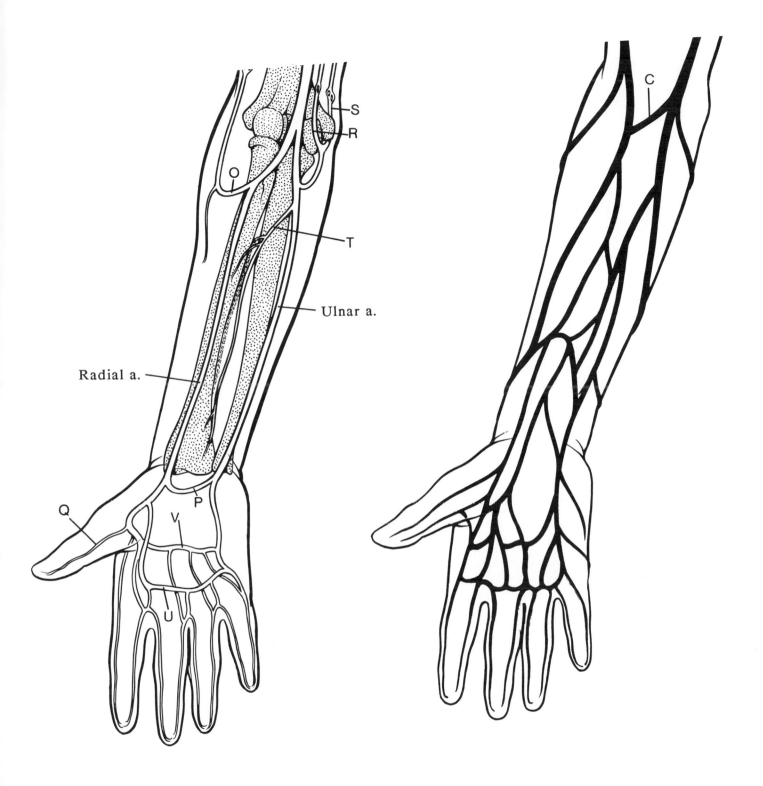

Fig. 4.7    Arterial Supply,
Forearm and Hand

Fig. 4.8    Superficial Venous Drainage,
Forearm and Hand

# CIRCULATORY SYSTEM OUTLINE

## UPPER LIMB

### ARTERIAL

I. **Subclavian (from aortic arch (L.); off bifurcation of brachiocephalic (Rt.); to lateral edge of first rib) (Figure 3.4)**

    A.   **Vertebral**

        Muscles of neck; spinal cord; brain

    B.   **Thyrocervical trunk**

        1.   Inferior thyroid

        2.   Suprascapular - clavicle and superior scapular area; anastomoses with scapular circumflex

        3.   Transverse cervical (descending scapular) - trapezius; levator scapula; rhomboids; supraspinatus; infraspinatus; subscapularis

    C.   **Internal thoracic**

II. **Axillary (continuation of subclavian; from lateral edge of first rib to the lower border of teres major)**

### Part One

Lateral border of first rib to superior border of pectoralis minor

    D.   **Supreme (highest) thoracic** - first and second intercostal spaces; pectoralis major and minor

### Part Two

Deep to the pectoralis minor

    E.   **Thoracocoacromial trunk** (clavicular, acromial, pectoral, and deltoid branches) - superior lateral thorax and acromial region of scapula; pectoral muscles and deltoid

    F.   **Lateral thoracic** (lateral mammary branches) - lateral thorax; pectoral muscles; serratus anterior; subscapularis

## Part Three

Inferior border of pectoralis minor to inferior border of teres major

    G.   **Subscapular**

        4.   Scapular circumflex - infraspinatus; teres major and minor; deltoid; long head of triceps; forms an anastomosis with the suprascapular

        5.   Thoracodorsal - lateral thoracic wall; latissimus dorsi; teres major

    II.   **Posterior humeral circumflex** - deltoid; shoulder joint

    I.   **Anterior humeral circumflex** - coracobrachialis; biceps brachii; shoulder joint

III.   **Brachial (continuation of axillary; from inferior border of teres major to cubital fossa)**

    J.   **Deep brachial (Profunda brachii)**

    K.   **Nutrient artery of humerus**

    L.   **Muscular branches**

    M.   **Superior ulnar collateral**

    N.   **Inferior ulnar collateral**

(The brachial artery and its branches supply all structures of the arm and participate in the anastomotic network around the elbow joint)

IV. **Radial (from bifurcation of brachial to hand) (Figures 3.4 and 4.7)**

Courses on lateral side of forearm, distributing to muscles on this side. Supplies most, but not all, extensors of wrist. Branches participate in anastomoses around elbow joint and carpals

    O.   **Radial recurrent**

    P.   **Carpal arch** - in an anastomosis with the ulnar artery

    Q.   **Princeps pollicis** - main supply to thumb

V. **Ulnar (bifurcates from brachial at same point as radial; continues to hand; accompanies ulnar nerve) (Figures 3.4 and 4.7)**

Courses on medial side of forearm supplying muscles on this side, including most flexors of wrist and hand. Branches participate in anastomoses around elbow joint and carpals

    R.   **Anterior ulnar recurrent**

    S.   **Posterior ulnar recurrent**

T.   **Common interosseous**

  6.   Anterior interosseous - courses on anterior surface of interosseous membrane supplying deep structures in the area

  7.   Posterior interosseous - courses on posterior surface of interosseous membrane supplying extensor muscles

## VI. Superficial and Deep Palmar Arches

After giving off the carpal arch the radial and ulnar arteries anastomose to form superficial and deep palmar arches in the hand. These arches, in turn, yield metacarpal and digital branches.

U.   **Superficial**

V.   **Deep**

## VENOUS

The deep veins of the upper limb generally accompany the arteries and are given the same name. Often these accompanying veins (venae comitantes) are paired, with the two veins united by numerous communicating veins.

In addition to a deep set of veins the upper limb also possesses a superficial set of veins (Figures 3.5 and 4.8). The key veins are:

A.   **Cephalic** - forms on the dorsal surface of the hand and ascends on the radial side of the limb; courses in the deltopectoral groove before passing deep to terminate in the axillary vein.

B.   **Basilic** - forms on the dorsal surface of the hand and ascends on the ulnar side of the limb; passes deep at about the mid-point of the arm and continues as the axillary vein at the lower border of the teres major.*

C.   **Medial Cubital** - a connecting vein between cephalic and basilic veins in front of the elbow joint; this vein is a common site for blood sampling and administration of anesthetics, saline solutions, etc.

*The basilic vein is usually described as continuing as the axillary vein at the lower border of the teres major. The brachial veins also terminate at about this point and may be described as joining with the basilic or the first part of the axillary. The axillary vein continues to the first rib, receiving drainage from the cephalic vein and deep veins in the area. At the first rib the axillary vein continues as the subclavian vein.

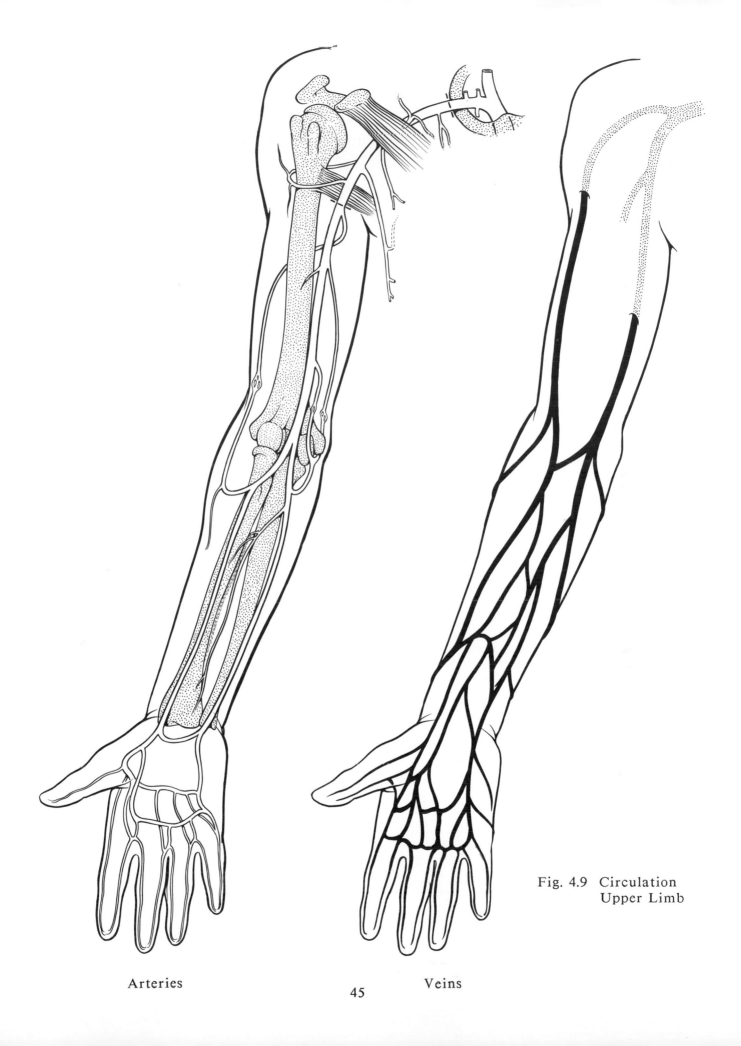

Fig. 4.9 Circulation
Upper Limb

Arteries

45

Veins

UNIT TWO: THORAX, ABDOMEN, PELVIS

## EXERCISE 5. VERTEBRAL COLUMN, SPINAL CORD, MUSCLES OF BACK

Study of the soft tissues of the back is enhanced when preceded by study of the vertebral column. The vertebral column (spine; spinal column) is the core structural unit of the trunk and plays a key role in movement and in the maintenance of the upright biped stance. The human column typically consists of 33 vertebrae: 7 cervical; 12 thoracic; 5 lumbar; 5 sacral (fused to form the sacrum); and 4 coccygeal (of which the first is often separate and the remaining three fused). Another important constituent of the vertebral column is the series of intervertebral disks that unite succeeding vertebral bodies from the second cervical vertebra to the lumbo-sacral junction.

I. **Examine individual specimens of cervical, thoracic, and lumbar vertebrae as well as sacrum and coccyx and find the following:**

A. **Cervical vertebrae (Figures 5.1 and 5.2)**

**Typical (C3 - C6) (Figure 5.1)**

1. Body

2. Spinous process

3. Transverse process

    a. Anterior tubercle

    b. Posterior tubercle

    c. Transverse foramen

4. Vertebral arch

    d. Pedicle

    e. Lamina

5. Vertebral foramen

6. Superior articular process and facet

7. Inferior articular process and facet

**Atypical (C1,C2) (Figure 5.2)**

**Atlas (C1) - lacks a body**

8. Anterior arch with fovea dentis

9. Posterior arch

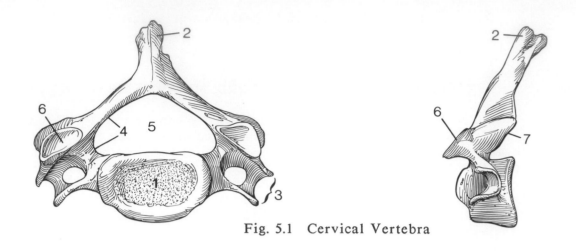

Fig. 5.1  Cervical Vertebra

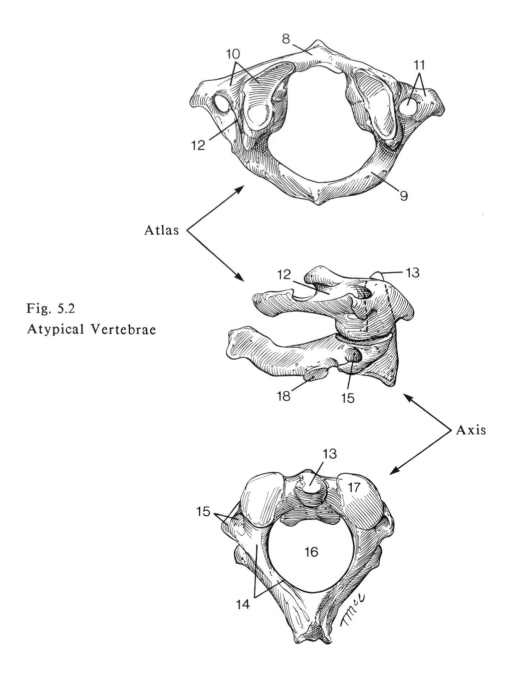

Atlas

Fig. 5.2
Atypical Vertebrae

Axis

10. Lateral mass with superior and inferior articular facets

11. Transverse process with transverse foramen

12. Sulcus for vertebral artery

### Axis (C2)

13. Dens (odontoid process)

14. Vertebral arch

15. Transverse process with transverse foramen

16. Vertebral foramen

17. Superior articular process and facet

18. Inferior articular process and facet

B. **Thoracic vertebrae (Figure 5.3)**

   1. Body, with costal facets

   2. Vertebral arch

     a. Pedicle

       (1) Superior vertebral notch

       (2) Inferior vertebral notch

     b. Lamina

   3. Spinous process

   4. Transverse process, with costal facet

   5. Vertebral foramen

   6. Superior articular process and facet

   7. Inferior articular process and facet

C. **Lumbar vertebrae (Figure 5.4)** - Lumbar vertebrae have specific characteristics based upon their role in support of the vertebral column.

   1. Body

   2. Vertebral arch

     a. Pedicle

       (1) Superior vertebral notch

49

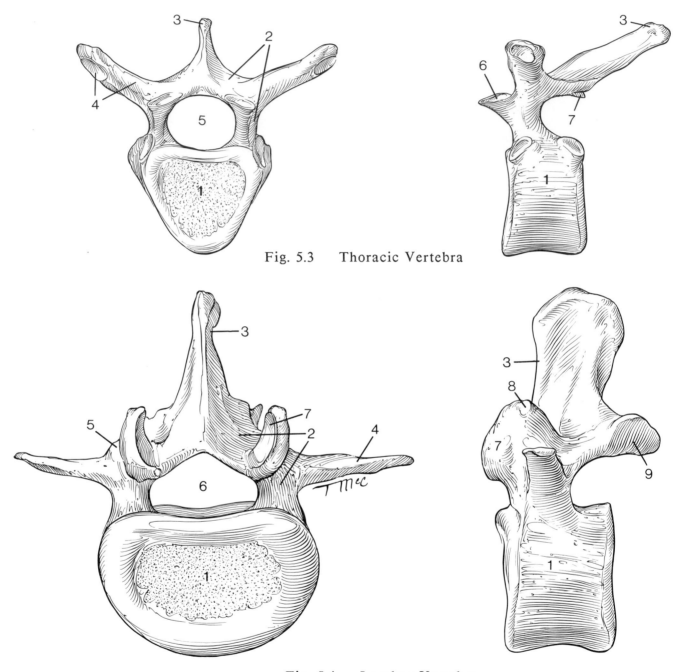

Fig. 5.3    Thoracic Vertebra

Fig. 5.4    Lumbar Vertebra

50

(2)    Inferior vertebral notch

    b.    Lamina

3.    Spinous process

4.    Transverse process - this is sometimes called a costal process because the distal portion represents a rudimentary rib

5.    Accessory process - found at the base of the transverse (costal) process

6.    Vertebral foramen

7.    Superior articular process and facet

8.    Mamillary process - found on the posterior surface of the superior articular process

9.    Inferior articular process and facet

D.   **Sacrum (Figures 5.5 and 5.6)**

1.    Superior articular process and facet

2.    Median crest

3.    Lateral mass with auricular surface for articulation with the ilium

4.    Sacral promontory

5.    Pelvic surface with foramina

6.    Dorsal surface with foramina

7.    Sacral canal

8.    Sacral cornu

9.    Sacral hiatus

E.   **Coccyx**

10.    Coccygeal cornu


## II. Muscles of the Back (Figure 5.7)

The superficial muscles of the back are muscles of the upper limb. These include the trapezius and latissimus dorsi most superficially and the rhomboids (major and minor) and levator scapula in a second layer.

The true muscles of the back are the erector spinae, a mass running from the sacrum to the skull and composed of three groups: iliocostalis, longissimus, and

51

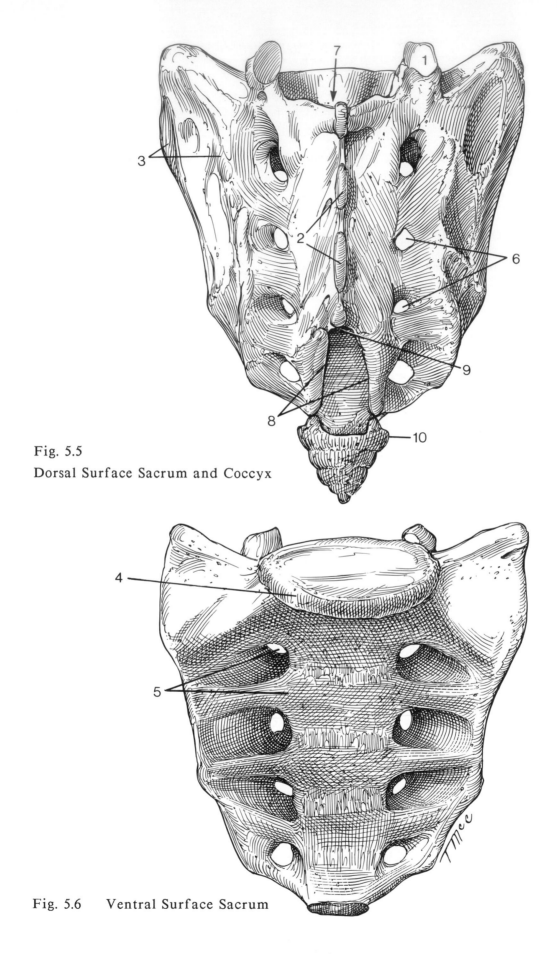

Fig. 5.5
Dorsal Surface Sacrum and Coccyx

Fig. 5.6    Ventral Surface Sacrum

spinalis. Each of these groups is in turn subdivided according to the region of the back upon which they function.

A.   **Iliocostalis** - This group has lumbar, thoracic, and cervical portions. It is the most lateral of the erector spinae and generally has attachments on transverse processes of vertebrae and the angles of the ribs.

B.   **Longissimus** - This muscle group has thoracic, cervical, and capital (head) portions. It is the middle group of the erector spinae and generally has attachments on the transverse processes of the vertebrae, with the distal attachment of the capital portion being the posterior margin of the mastoid bone.

C.   **Spinalis** - This is the most medial of the erector spinae, with attachments on the spinous processes. Thoracic and cervical portions of this muscle are usually described.

In the neck muscles are adapted in size and orientation to support the weight of the head and to assist in moving the head.

The important muscles of the neck include:

D.   **Splenius capitis**

E.   **Semispinalis capitis**

F.   **Spinalis capitis**

What is the general function of the erector spinae?

Given this, how would you describe the relationship of proximal and distal attachments of these muscles?

What is the nerve supply of the erector spinae and does this supply differ in any way from that of the upper limb muscles?

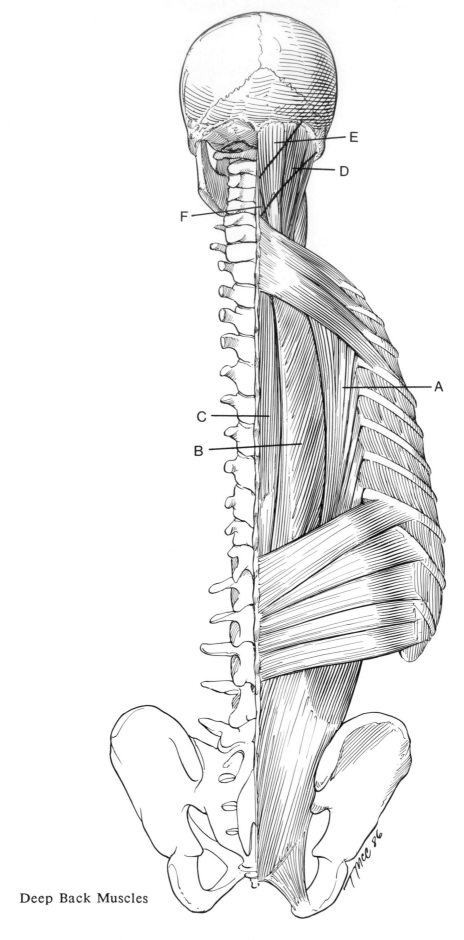

Fig. 5.7    Deep Back Muscles

## III. Vertebral Canal and Spinal Cord (Figures 5.8 and 5.9)

The spinal cord, protected by its meningeal coverings, lies within the vertebral canal. (In dissection, these parts can be observed by removing the erector spinae in the lumbar region and performing a laminectomy.) Figure 5.8 shows features of these structures.

A. The ligamentum flavum pass from lamina to lamina on the deep surface of the lamina.

B. Considerable amounts of epidural fat surround the spinal cord. Within this fat exists the vertebral plexus of veins. The fat provides some insulation and protection while the veins form a system running the length of the column and capable of carrying considerable amounts of blood in certain situations.

C. The dura mater (L., tough mother) lies beneath the epidural fat. This grayish-colored membrane surrounds the entire central nervous system.

D. The posterior longitudinal ligament passes along the posterior surface of the vertebral bodies. (In dissection, this can be seen if the spinal cord is moved gently to one side with a probe.)

The following structures are apparent after the dura mater is split mid-dorsally for the length of the exposed area (Figures 5.8 and 5.9).

E. **Arachnoid mater**

F. **Conus medullaris**

G. **Cauda equina**

H. **Filum terminale**

I. **Pia mater** - this is in the form of denticulate ligaments

J. **Dorsal and ventral rootlets of spinal nerves**

K. **Ventral rootlets of spinal nerves**

L. **Dorsal root ganglion**

If you are dissecting a cadaver, turn your attention to the dorsal and ventral rootlets of one spinal nerve. Identify dorsal (sensory) rootlets and ventral (motor) rootlets. Trace these distally to the exit of the nerve from the vertebral canal. This point of exit is an intervertebral foramen, which contains a dorsal root ganglion. The dura mater surrounding the spinal cord is continuous over the spinal nerves through the intervertebral foramina, after which it fuses with their epineurial sheaths.

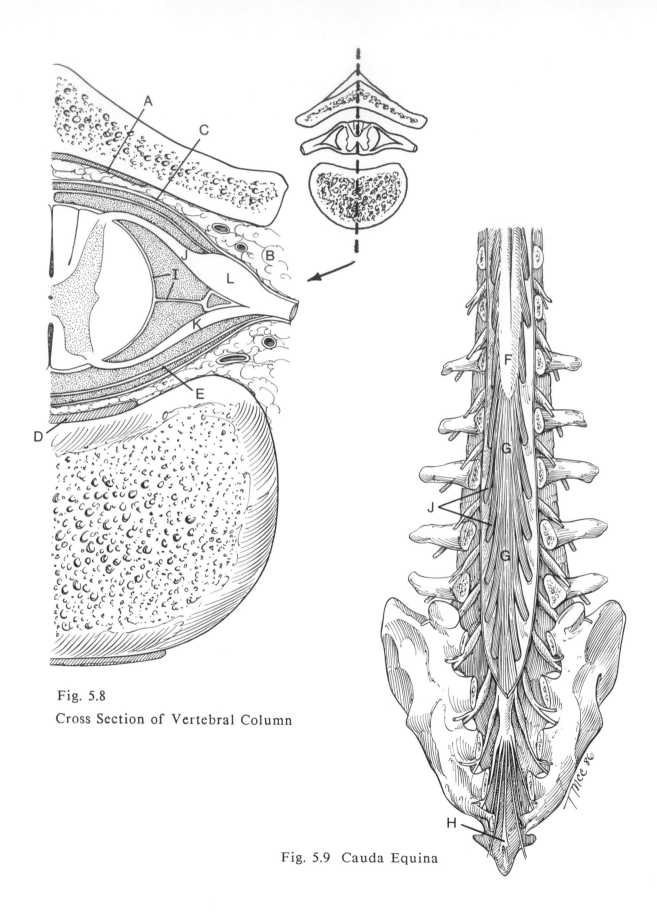

Fig. 5.8

Cross Section of Vertebral Column

Fig. 5.9  Cauda Equina

**FOR REVIEW AND THOUGHT**

Discuss with your laboratory/study partners the significance of the region you have just studied. Be able to answer the following questions.

1. What processes brought about the formation of the cauda equina and surrounding sub-arachnoid space?

2. What is the significance of this region for diagnostic and anesthetic procedures?

# NOTES

# EXERCISE 6. THORACIC WALL AND CONTENTS

The thoracic wall is composed of vertebral column (already studied), sternum, ribs, and associated muscles. The area between a pair of ribs is an intercostal space and there are, therefore, eleven such spaces on each side of the thorax. In the human each intercostal space typically contains three muscles, arranged in incomplete layers, and a neurovascular supply.

## I. Thoracic Wall (Figures 6.1 - 6.5)

A. **Ribs and Sternum** - Use a skeleton to study the bony thorax.

The twelve pair of ribs are often described as "true" (articulating with a vertebra posteriorly and, via a costal cartilage, with the sternum anteriorly; ribs 1-7) and "false" (articulating posteriorly with a vertebra but anteriorly articulating with the costal cartilage of the rib above, as with ribs 8-10, or remaining free anteriorly, as with ribs 11 and 12).

**Typical rib** (Figure 6.1) Each typical rib has a vertebral and sternal extremity with an intervening body. Label the following portions of a typical rib on Figure 6.1.

1. Head - with an articular surface divided into two parts by a small ridge; these two articular areas are called demifacets

2. Neck - about one inch in length and located just lateral to the head

3. Tubercle - found at the junction of the neck and body; possesses an articular facet

4. Angle - an oblique ridge lateral to the tubercle on the external surface

5. Costal groove - on the internal surface of the rib, along and just superior to the inferior border

**Atypical ribs** (Figure 6.2)

6. First rib - This rib is the shortest and has the greatest curvature. It is flattened in a plane different from the other ribs so there are superior and inferior surfaces. Specific characteristics of the first rib are:

   a. The head has no division of its articular facet

   b. The tubercle is thick and prominent

   c. No angle is present

   d. The superior surface shows two shallow grooves for the subclavian artery and vein, with an intervening tubercle for the attachment of the anterior scalene muscle

59

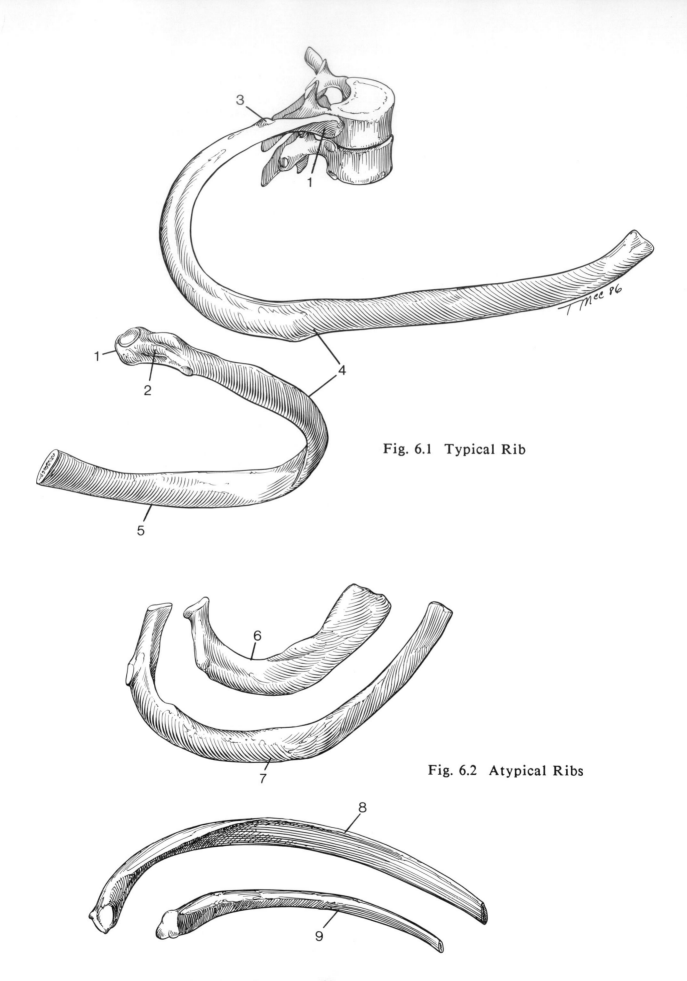

Fig. 6.1  Typical Rib

Fig. 6.2  Atypical Ribs

60

e. No costal groove is present

7. Second rib - This rib is intermediate in form to the first rib and a typical rib; it possesses a curvature similar to the first rib but is not quite as flattened; the angle is slight and close to the tubercle

8. Eleventh rib

9. Twelfth rib

The eleventh and twelfth ribs possess several characteristics

a. A single articular facet on the head

b. A lack of either a neck or tubercle

c. Eleventh has a very shallow costal groove and the twelfth has none

With what does(do) the articular facet(s) on the head of the rib articulate?




With what do the tubercular facets articulate?




Describe the articulation of a typical rib to the vertebral column!




**Sternum** (Figure 6.3) - The sternum is described in three parts, the manubrium, body, and xiphoid process.

10. Manubrium - the most cephalic portion of the sternum; the jugular notch is found on the superior surface, on either side of which is an articular surface for the clavicle; just inferior to this is an area for articulation with the first rib

11. Body - the largest portion of the sternum; articulates with the third through seventh costal cartilages

12. Xiphoid process - the most caudal portion of the sternum; it may be bifid; articulates partially with the seventh rib

**Sternal angle** (of Lewis) - A prominent ridge is usually present at the junction of the manubrium and the body. This ridge is palpable and is an important anatomical landmark because it indicates the level of the articulation of the second rib to the sternum.

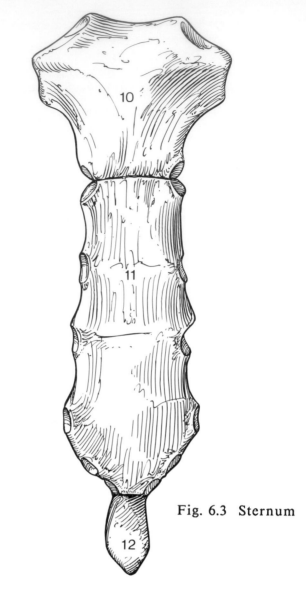

Fig. 6.3  Sternum

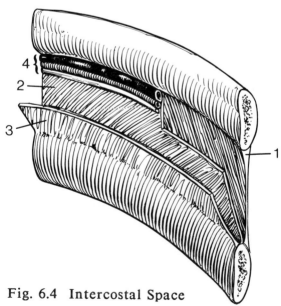

Fig. 6.4  Intercostal Space

B. **Intercostal Muscles and Vessels (Figures 6.4 and 6.5)**

1. The fibers of the external intercostal muscle can be seen in the mid-lateral portion of an intercostal space. These fibers course inferiorly and medially. In the more inferior intercostal spaces this muscle is continuous with the external oblique muscle of the abdominal wall.

2. When a portion of the external intercostal is removed, the underlying internal intercostal muscle is exposed. The fibers of this muscle pass superiorly and medially.

3. The deepest muscle layer in an intercostal space is the innermost intercostal. The fibers of this muscle course in the same direction as those of the internal intercostal, and between these two layers are the intercostal nerve and vessels.

4. The nerve and vessels are usually found just inferior to the superior rib and are arranged in the order of vein, artery, and nerve - VAN.

5. On the inner surface of the thoracic cage is the transverse thoracis, a thin layer of muscle arising from the deep surface of the sternum and extending cranially and laterally to attach to the costal cartilages of the second to sixth ribs (Figure 6.5).

6. The internal thoracic vessels course anterior to the transverse thoracis, between it and the costal cartilages and internal intercostals. If the transverse thoracis is cut along its sternal attachment, the interal thoracic artery and vein may be seen giving off anterior intercostal branches (Figure 6.5).

From what vessel is the internal thoracic artery a branch?

_____

What are the two terminal branches of the internal thoracic artery and what is their distribution? _____

_____ and _____

_____.

Intercostal spaces are also supplied by posterior intercostal arteries. From what vessel do such posterior intercostal arteries arise? _____

_____

Parietal pleura, a glistening layer of connective tissue lining the inside of the thoracic wall, is found deep to the innermost intercostal muscles. This layer is best seen from the inside of the thorax after removal of the ribs. The parietal pleura is continuous with the visceral pleura at the root of the lung (Figure 6.8).

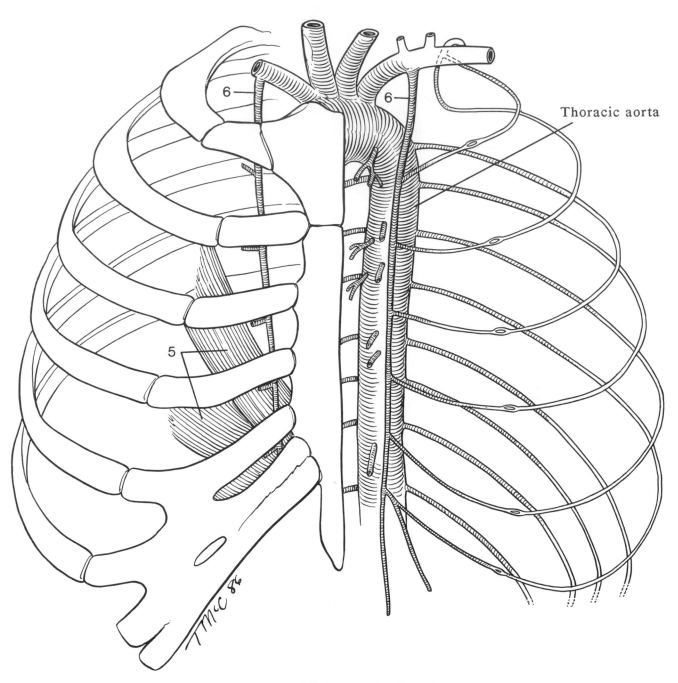

Fig. 6.5  Thoracic Vessels

## II. Thoracic Cavity and Lungs (Figures 6.6 - 6.9)

With the thoracic cage removed the thoracic cavity is now exposed. "Observe and appreciate" the relationship of various structures in the thorax. Find the following on Figures 6.6 through 6.8.

A. **Heart** (in pericardial sac)

B. **Lungs**

C. **Trachea**

D. **Esophagus**

E. **Azygos vein** (arching above the right primary bronchus to empty into the superior vena cava)

F. **Aortic arch**

The area between the lungs, containing the heart and other structures, is the mediastinum (Figure 6.6).

G. **Phrenic nerves.** These nerves arise from cervical spinal levels 3-5 and innervate the diaphragm. What might account for such a seeming anomaly? In their course to the diaphragm these nerves often adhere to the fibrous pericardium (Figure 6.7).

H. **Cranial Nerve X** (the vagus nerve). Vagus is a Latin word meaning "wandering," and that is exactly what this nerve and its branches do in supplying parasympathetic innervation to the neck, thorax, and abdomen. The right vagus lies posterior to the right brachiocephalic vein and anterior to the right subclavian artery. The left vagus is found anterior to the arch of the aorta. Both vagi give rise to recurrent laryngeal nerves, which loop around the subclavian artery (right) and aortic arch (left) and ascend between the trachea and esophagus to reach the larynx. After giving off branches to the cardiac plexus, both vagi pass posterior to the pulmonary vessels and bronchi to form an esophageal plexus prior to passing through the diaphragm to reach the abdomen (Figure 6.7).

I. **Visceral Pleura** (Figure 6.8). Visceral pleura is continuous at the root of the lung with the parietal pleura lining the thoracic wall. The right lung has three lobes and the left lung has two lobes, divided by observable fissures. The visceral pleura is continuous within these fissures.

J. **Parietal Pleura**

K. **Pleural Cavity** - This is a potential space between the visceral and parietal pleura.

Figure 6.7 is a lateral view of the thorax with the right lung removed, showing the cut surfaces of the bronchus and vessels, while Figure 6.9 shows details of the tracheal bifurcation.

L. **Right Primary Bronchus**

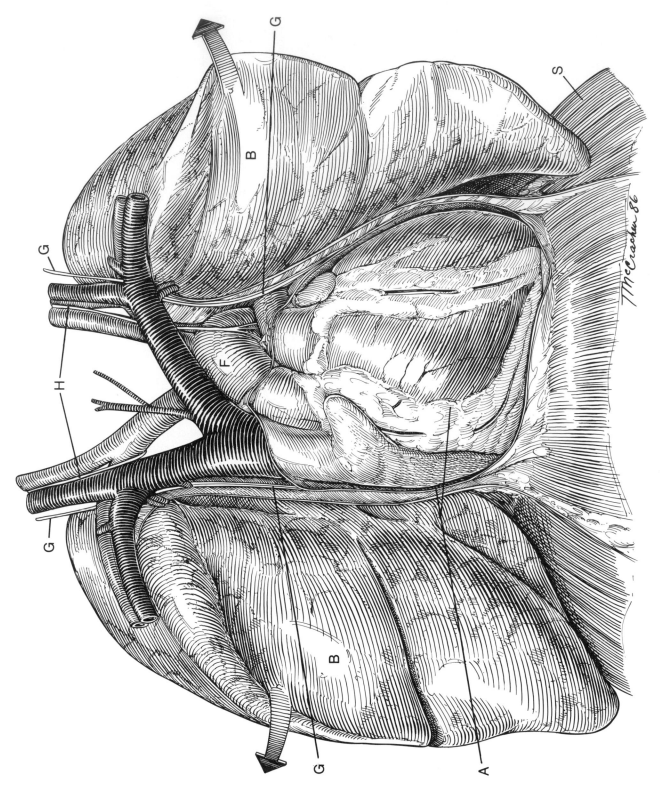

Fig. 6.6 Thoracic Viscera

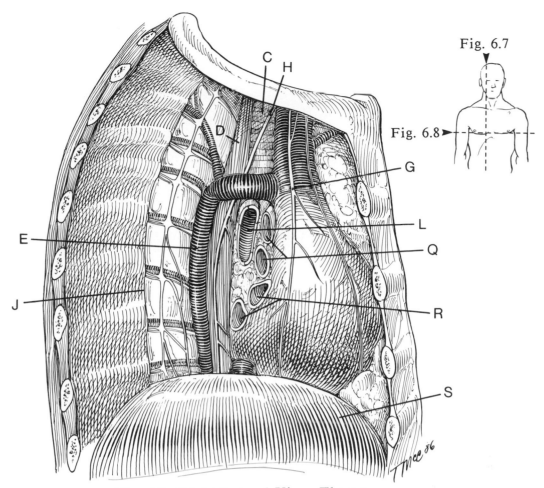

Fig. 6.7 Right Lateral View, Thorax

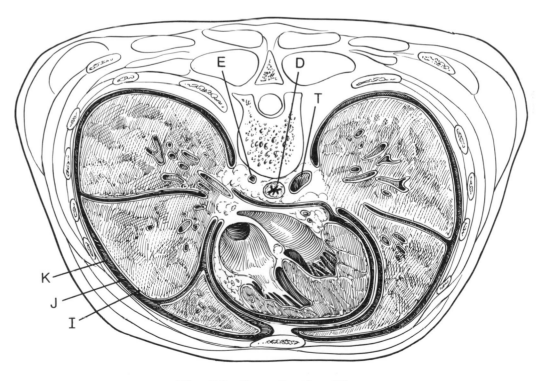

Fig. 6.8 Cross Section, Thorax

M.   **Left Primary Bronchus**

N.   **Right Secondary Bronchi**

O.   **Left Secondary Bronchi**

P.   **Carina**

Q.   **Pulmonary Arteries**

R.   **Pulmonary Veins**

S.   **Diaphragm**

T.   **Thoracic Aorta**

Note that the right primary bronchus branches at a less acute angle than the left. On the inferior boundary of the bifurcation is a prominent ridge, the carina. The carina is significant because the mucous membrane of this area is richly supplied with nerves that promote the cough reflex.

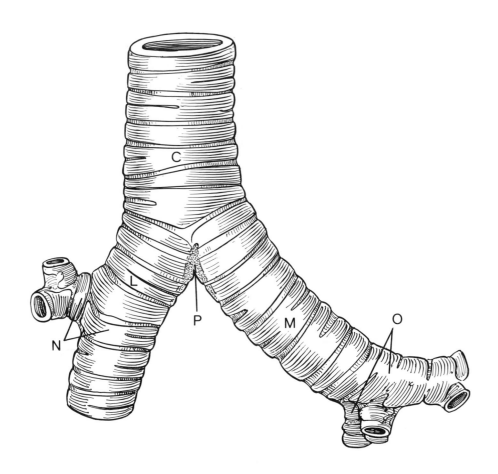

Fig. 6.9   Tracheal Bifurcation

## FOR REVIEW AND THOUGHT

Be sure you understand the concept of parietal and visceral pleura, for the same concept will hold true in the abdomen when dealing with peritoneum. Portions of the parietal pleura are given additional descriptive names dependent upon the region of the thoracic cavity: thus diaphragmatic, costal, and mediastinal pleurae are all terms to describe specific portions of the parietal pleura. Look again at the diaphragm. This muscle serves as a physical boundary between the thorax and abdomen. What structures do you see passing through this boundary? **LIST THEM!**

From what has been said about the primary bronchi, into which bronchus would you expect an aspirated object to pass?

Given its innervation, where might you expect pain from the diaphragm to be referred?

69

# EXERCISE 7. HEART AND GREAT VESSELS

The heart is a four-chambered muscular pump which, postnatally, is divisible into pulmonary and systemic circuits (Figure 7.1). The pulmonary portion of the heart (right chambers) pumps oxygen-deficient blood to the lungs while the systemic portion (left chambers) pumps oxygen-enriched blood to the entire body. Keep this basic premise clearly in mind and both prenatal and postnatal heart function will make sense, as will the changes in circulation occurring at, and shortly after, birth. Figures 7.1 and 7.2 are conceptual representations of the postnatal circulation, with oxygen-rich blood depicted in clear vessels and oxygen-deficient blood in dark vessels.

When viewed anteriorly, portions of all chambers of the heart are visible. The bulk of the anterior surface, however, is formed by the right ventricle. When the heart is observed in situ with its surrounding pericardium, the pericardium continues for some distance onto the great vessels.

I.   Identify the following structures in Figures 7.3 - 7.5, which show the heart with the pericardium removed and the great vessels cut some distance away from the heart:

   A.   **Brachiocephalic veins**

   B.   **Superior vena cava**

   C.   **Inferior vena cava**

   D.   **Pulmonary trunk and arteries**

   E.   **Pulmonary veins**

   F.   **Aortic arch**

   G.   **Brachiocephalic trunk**

   H.   **Common carotid arteries**

   I.   **Subclavian arteries**

Orientation to the chambers of the heart is facilitated by finding the superior and inferior venae cavae entering the right atrium. Do so, then find the remaining chambers of the heart.

   J.   **Right atrium with auricle**

   K.   **Right ventricle**

   L.   **Left atrium with auricle**

   M.   **Left ventricle**

   N.   **Apex of the heart** - inferior tip of left ventricle

The coronary arteries are found on the surface of the heart but are often obscured by fat. The same is true of the coronary sinus, the main venous drainage of the

71

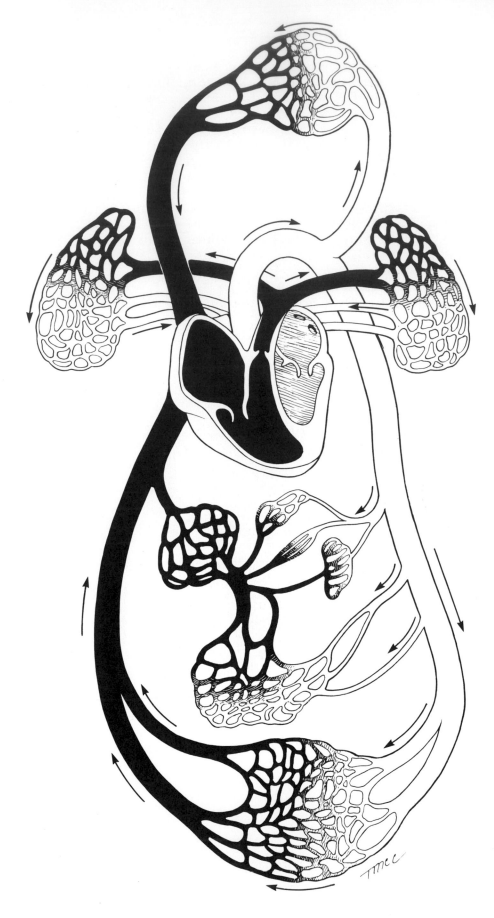

Fig. 7.1  Schematic Circulatory System

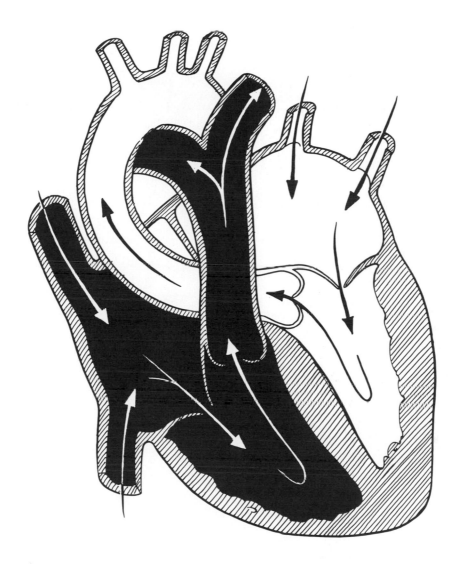

Fig. 7.2  Blood Flow Through Heart

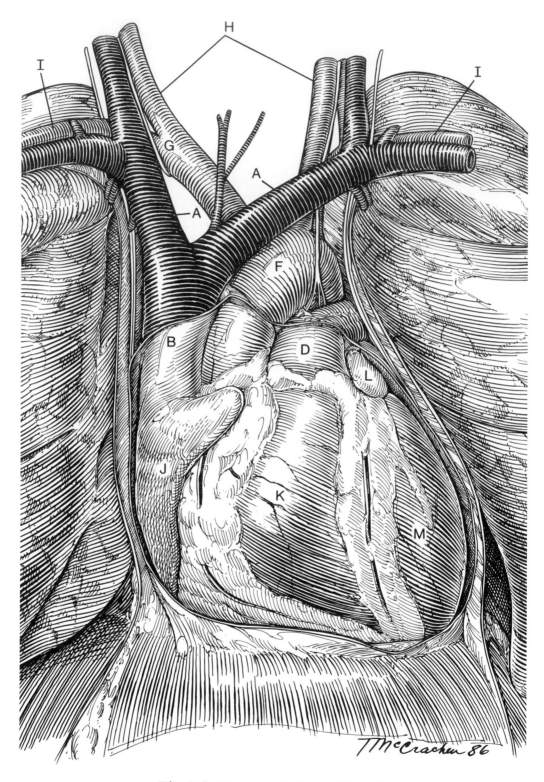

Fig. 7.3  Heart and Great Vessels

heart.   The coronary arteries (Figures 7.4 and 7.5) arise from the base of the ascending aorta.   The right coronary artery courses in the groove between the right atrium and right ventricle to the posterior aspect of the heart.   As this vessel reaches the inferior margin of the right ventricle it gives off the marginal artery, and continues posteriorly with its main terminal branch being the posterior interventricular artery.   The left coronary artery is found between the left atrium and the pulmonary trunk.   This vessel is very short, dividing into the circumflex and anterior interventricular arteries.   The circumflex coronary artery courses in the groove between the left atrium and ventricle to the posterior aspect of the heart where it anastomoses with a branch of the right coronary artery.   The anterior interventricular artery courses on the anterior surface of the heart between the ventricles and passes over the apex of the heart to ascend posteriorly and anastomose with the posterior interventricular artery.

The great cardiac vein is found accompanying the anterior interventricular artery and will form the coronary sinus.   The middle cardiac vein accompanies the posterior interventricular artery and empties into the coronary sinus.   The coronary sinus, in turn, empties into the right atrium.   Anterior cardiac veins, draining the right atrium and ventricle, typically empty into the right atrium independent of the coronary sinus.

O.   **Right coronary artery**

P.   **Marginal artery**

Q.   **Posterior interventricular artery**

R.   **Left coronary artery**

S.   **Circumflex artery**

T.   **Anterior interventricular artery**

U.   **Great cardiac vein**

V.   **Middle cardiac vein**

W.   **Anterior cardiac veins**

X.   **Coronary sinus**

II.   When the chambers of the heart are incised and cleaned of blood the following structures are seen (Figures 7.6 and 7.7).

A.   **Opening of the coronary sinus**

B.   **Tricuspid valve**

C.   **Papillary muscles**

D.   **Chordae tendinae**

E.   **Pulmonary trunk with semi-lunar valves**

75

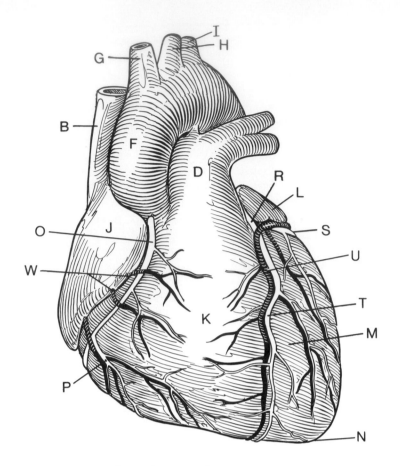

Fig. 7.4  Anterior Heart

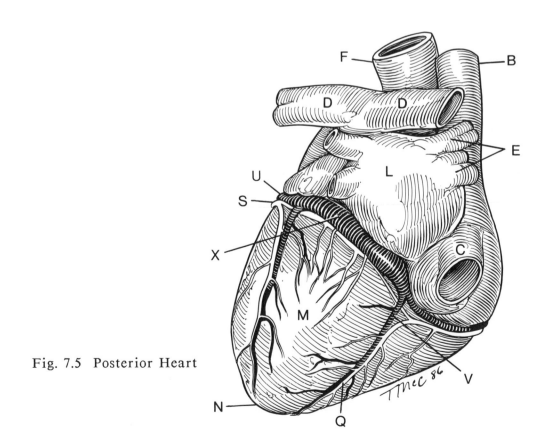

Fig. 7.5  Posterior Heart

F. **Bicuspid (Mitral) valve**

G. **Ascending aorta with semi-lunar valves**

H. **Sinuses of the semi-lunar valves**

III. **Remnants of Pre-natal Circulation**

Two vestiges of the prenatal circulation remain postnatally: the fossa ovalis and the ligamentum arteriosum. The fossa ovalis was the foramen ovale, connecting the right and left atria. The ligamentum arteriosum was the ductus arteriosus, connecting the pulmonary trunk with the aortic arch. Find these on Figures 7.6 and 7.7.

I. **Fossa ovalis**

J. **Ligamentum arteriosum**

## FOR REVIEW AND THOUGHT

Discuss with a study partner the differences between pre- and postnatal circulation from a functional viewpoint. What purpose did the foramen ovale and ductus arteriosus serve? Why was the ductus arteriosus situated downstream from the vessels to the head and upper limb arising from the aorta?

Describe the action of the atrio-ventricular valves and the roles played by papillary muscles and chordae tendinae! Compare this with the action of the semi-lunar valves.

Attempt to trace a sample of blood from the skin of the left thumb through the venous drainage of the upper limb, heart, and arterial supply, to the muscles of the right thumb!

## NOTES

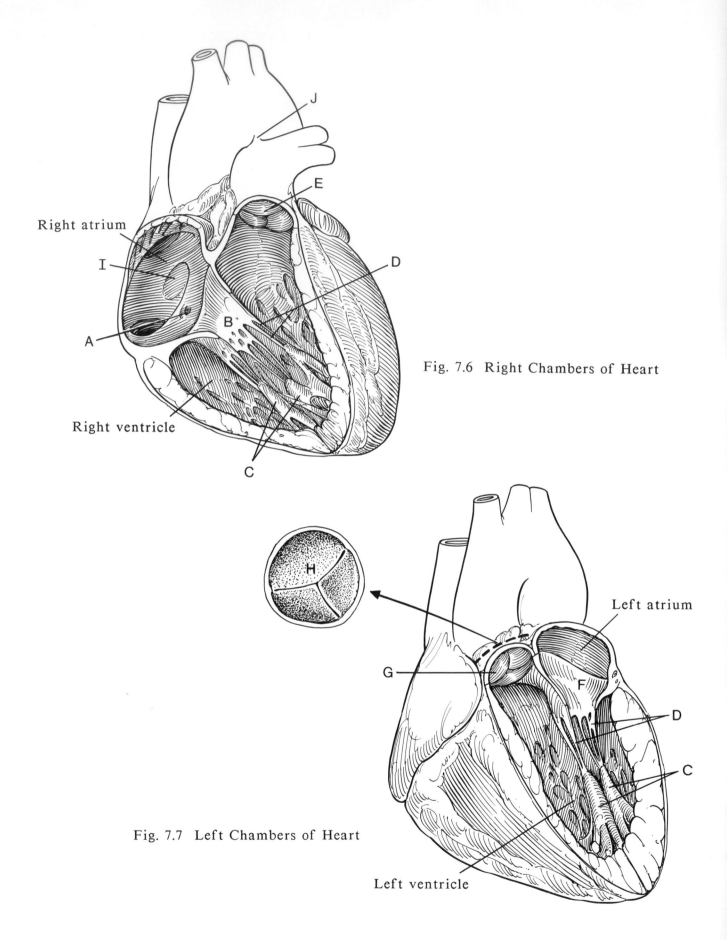

Right atrium

I

A

Right ventricle

E

D

B

C

Fig. 7.6  Right Chambers of Heart

J

H

Left atrium

G

F

D

C

Left ventricle

Fig. 7.7  Left Chambers of Heart

# EXERCISE 8.  ABDOMINAL WALL; ABDOMINAL AND PELVIC CONTENTS

The abdominal wall is composed of layered muscles whose fibers run in different directions, much like the intercostal muscles. As you study the muscles of the abdominal wall, observe and appreciate the direction in which the muscle fibers course.

## I.  Abdominal Muscles (Figures 8.1 and 8.2)

### A.  Rectus abdominus

The "straight" abdominal muscles run longitudinally on each side of a tough midline structure, the linea alba. The proximal attachment of the rectus abdominus is the pubic crest. What is the distal attachment?

DA -

The rectus abdominus is enveloped by the aponeuroses of the external and internal oblique muscles and the transverse abdominus as they pass toward their distal attachment on the linea alba. This envelope is known as the rectus sheath.

### B.  External oblique

The fibers of this muscle pass inferiorly and medially from their proximal attachment on the lower 8 ribs and attach distally into the linea alba via an aponeurosis that passes anterior to the rectus abdominus.

### C.  Internal oblique

This muscle takes proximal attachment from the lateral half of the inguinal ligament, the anterior portion of the iliac crest, and the thoracolumbar fascia. Its fibers pass superiorly and medially to attach to ribs 9-12 and via an aponeurosis into the linea alba. This distal attachment is unique and more will be said of it below.

### D.  Transverse abdominus

This is the deepest of the three muscle layers. It has a similar proximal attachment as the internal oblique and a distal aponeurotic attachment into the linea alba.

On the deep surface of the rectus abdominus approximately midway between the umbilicus and pubic crest is the arcuate line. This line is a landmark indicating an abrupt change in the composition of the anterior and posterior layers of the rectus sheath. Above this line the aponeurosis of the internal oblique splits to pass both anteriorly and posteriorly to the rectus abdominus, and that of the transverse abdominus passes posteriorly. Below this line all of these aponeuroses pass anterior to the rectus abdominus, leaving only the transversalis fascia on the posterior wall of the muscle.

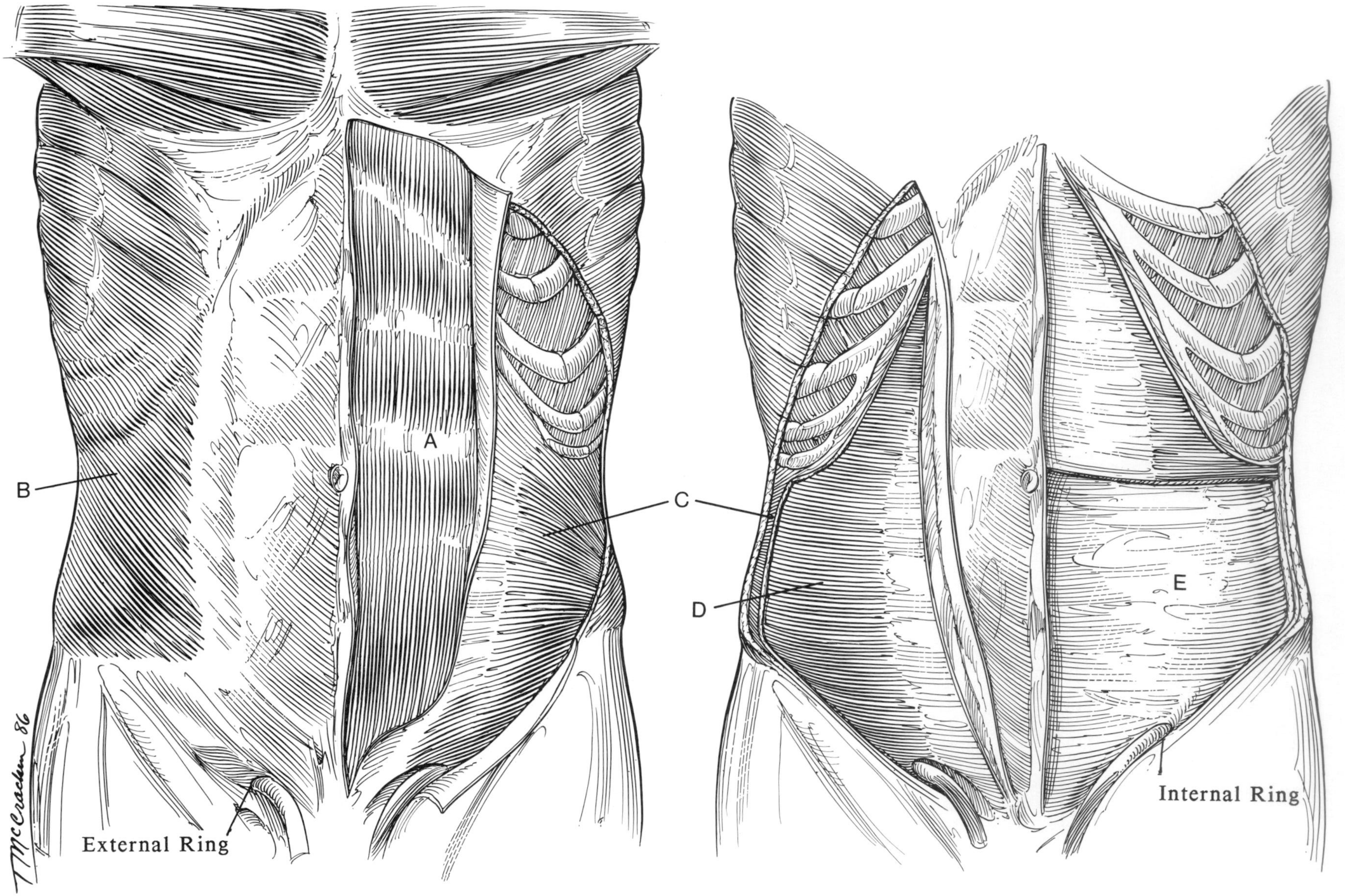

Fig. 8.2 Deep

Abdominal Wall

Fig. 8.1 Superficial

80

Between the internal oblique and transverse abdominus is the segmental nerve supply of the abdominal wall. How is this similar to the situation in the thoracic wall?

This segmental innervation is from levels T7 through L1 with T10 supplying the area around the umbilicus. Given this, develop a picture of the innervation of the abdominal wall.

E. **Transversalis fascia**

This thin layer of fascia is found immediately deep to the transverse abdominus.

II. **Peritoneum (Figure 8.3)**

The deepest layer of the abdominal wall is the parietal peritoneum. As was the case in the pleural cavities, the abdominal cavity is possessed of both visceral and parietal peritoneum. Figure 8.3 presents a schematic interpretation of the peritoneum. Parietal peritoneum lines the body wall and dorsally is reflected onto the viscera of the gastrointestinal tract as a double layer. This double layer of peritoneum is a mesentery and it is through such a mesentery that the nerves and vascular supply reach the viscera. The layer of peritoneum intimately covering the viscera is known as visceral peritoneum. Label the following on Figure 8.3.

A. **Parietal peritoneum**

B. **Visceral peritoneum**

C. **Mesentery**

Some organs (the kidneys are represented in Figure 8.3) do not have a mesentery and are described as being retroperitoneal. In all cases this does not literally mean "behind the peritoneum," but means "without a mesentery." As you study and learn the various organs of the abdomen and pelvis, decide whether they are with or without a mesentery.

III. **Abdominal Contents (Figures 8.4 and 8.5)** - When the abdominal wall has been opened, the first structure encountered will be the greater omentum, an apron-like double fold of peritoneum hanging down over the intestines from the inferior border of the stomach. Locate the following structures of the gastrointestinal tract and list whether or not they have a mesentery.

A. **Esophagus**

B. **Stomach**

    1. Cardiac sphincter

    2. Fundus

    3. Pyloric sphincter

C. **Duodenum**

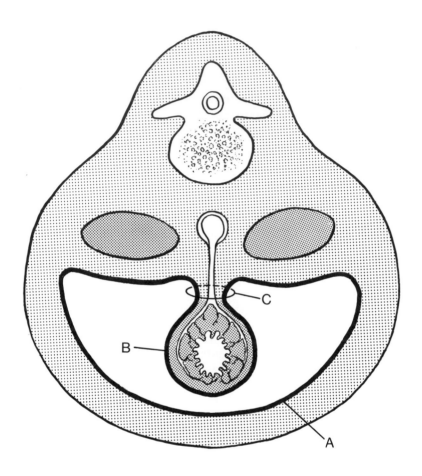

Fig. 8.3  Schematic of Peritoneal Cavity

D. Jejunum

E. Ileum

F. Cecum

G. Vermiform appendix

H. Colon - Ascending, transverse, descending

Now find the glands associated with the gastrointestinal tract (Figure 8.5).

I. Liver

J. Hepatic bile duct

K. Gallbladder

L. Cystic bile duct

M. Common bile duct

N. Pancreas

O. Pancreatic duct

IV. Other Abdominal Structures (Figure 8.6)

A. Inferior phrenic artery

B. Celiac trunk

C. Superior mesenteric artery

D. Inferior mesenteric artery

E. Renal artery

F. Gonadal arteries

G. Lumbar arteries

H. Bifurcation of aorta

I. Hepatic veins

J. Renal vein

K. Gonadal veins

L. Adrenal gland

M. Kidney

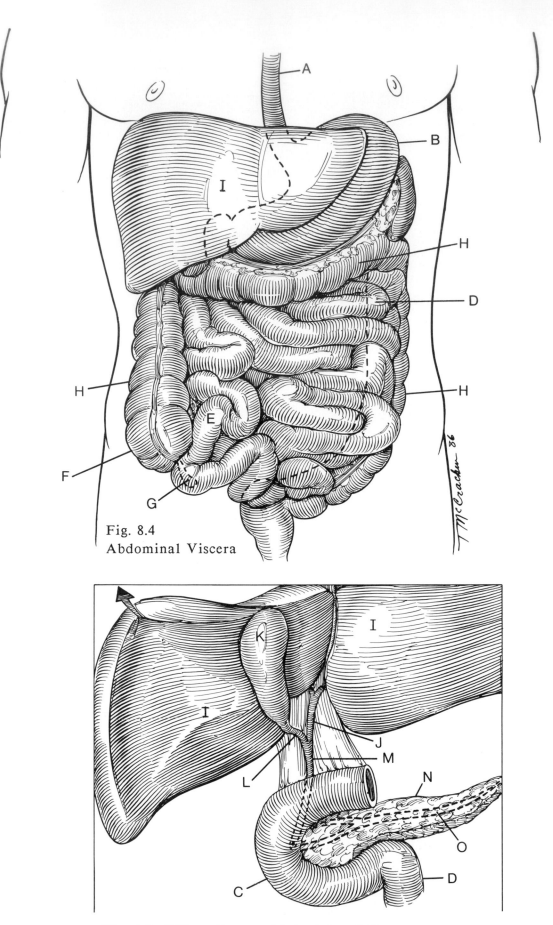

Fig. 8.4
Abdominal Viscera

Fig. 8.5 Biliary System (right lobe of liver retracted)

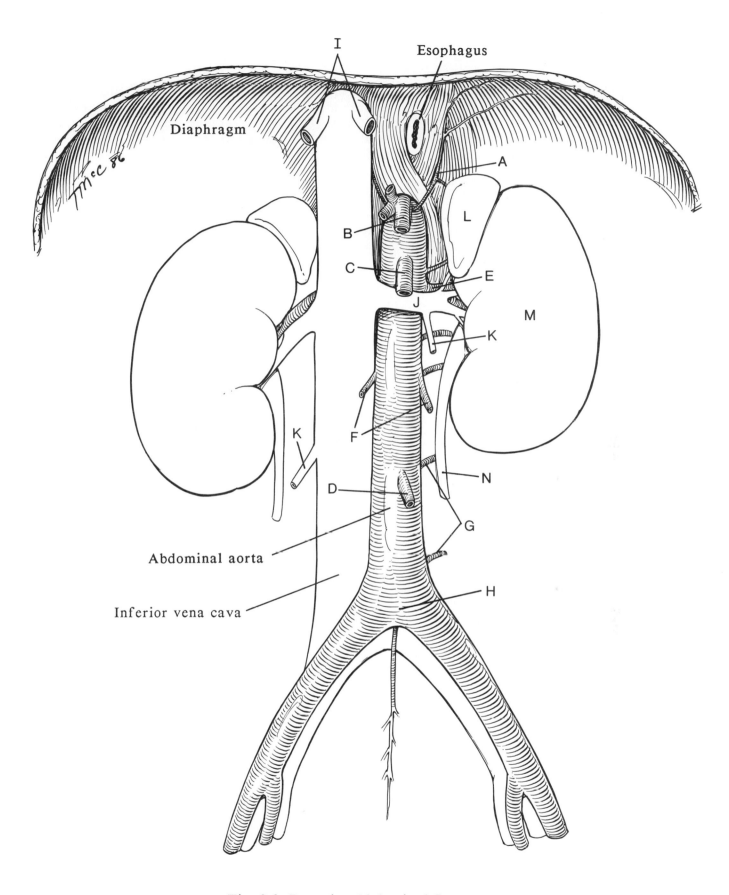

Fig. 8.6 Posterior Abdominal Structures

N.   Ureter

## V. Pelvic Viscera

The pelvic cavity is merely an extension of the abdominal cavity.  The true pelvis is considered that area below the pelvic inlet while the area above the inlet is considered the abdomen and is sometimes referred to as the false pelvis.  Some abdominal structures continue into the pelvis.  A good example of this is the sigmoid colon, which leaves the abdomen by curling over the pelvic brim to become the rectum.  Since both are portions of the gastrointestinal tract, note whether or not they possess a mesentery.

Also passing from abdomen to pelvis are the ureters, connecting the kidneys (abdominal) with the urinary bladder (pelvic).  Find the following structures in the lower abdomen and pelvis (Figure 8.7).

A.   **Abdominal aorta**

B.   **Inferior vena cava**

C.   **Common iliac artery**

D.   **External iliac artery**

E.   **Internal iliac artery**

The aorta splits into paired common iliac arteries at what vertebral level? _____ Each common iliac then branches into external and internal branches. To where are each of these branches destined to go? _____

In the female identify the following structures (Figure 8.8).

A.   **Ovary**

B.   **Body of uterus**

C.   **Uterine (Fallopian) tube**

D.   **Cervix of uterus**

E.   **Vagina**

F.   **Anterior fornix of vagina**

G.   **Posterior fornix of vagina**

H.   **Urinary bladder**

I.   **Urethra**

J.   **Rectum**

K.   **Rectouterine pouch**

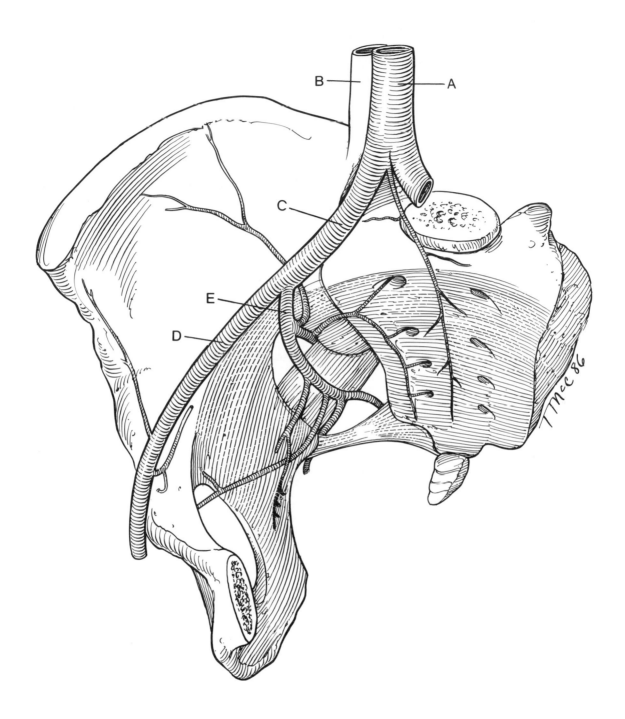

Fig. 8.7    Arterial Supply to Pelvis

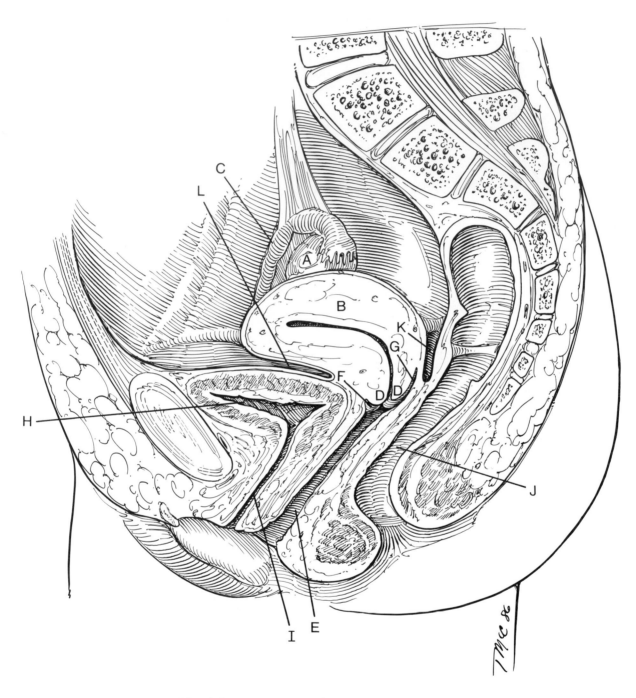

Fig. 8.8  Female Pelvis:  Mid-sagittal View

L.  **Vesicouterine pouch**

Note the relationship of the ureters to the uterine arteries and to the cervix of the uterus.

In the male identify the following structures (Figure 8.9).

A.  **Testis**

B.  **Epididymis**

C.  **Vas deferens**

D.  **Urinary bladder**

E.  **Prostate gland**

F.  **Urethra**

G.  **Penis**

H.  **Seminal vesicle**

I.  **Ejaculatory duct**

J.  **Scrotum**

K.  **Rectum**

L.  **Rectovesical pouch**

The reproductive organs (testes, ovaries) develop retroperitoneally in the supero-lateral abdomen, near the kidneys.  In the seventh to ninth fetal months these organs descend to their adult position.  In the case of the testes such position is in the scrotum.  In their passage through the abdominal wall to the scrotum the testes carry the vas deferens, testicular artery and vein, nerve supply, and lymphatics with them (Figure 8.10).  These structures, together with the layers of the abdominal wall picked up during passage, are known as the spermatic cord.

The ovaries descend to the pelvis, dragging the ovarian artery and vein, nerve supply, and lymphatics with them, but do not pass through the abdominal wall (Figure 8.11).  Structures known as the round ligaments, which helped guide the ovaries on their descent, do pass through the abdominal wall to reach the labia majora, where they dissipate in fibrous strands.  Label the structures just described in Figures 8.10 and 8.11

_____

_____

_____

_____

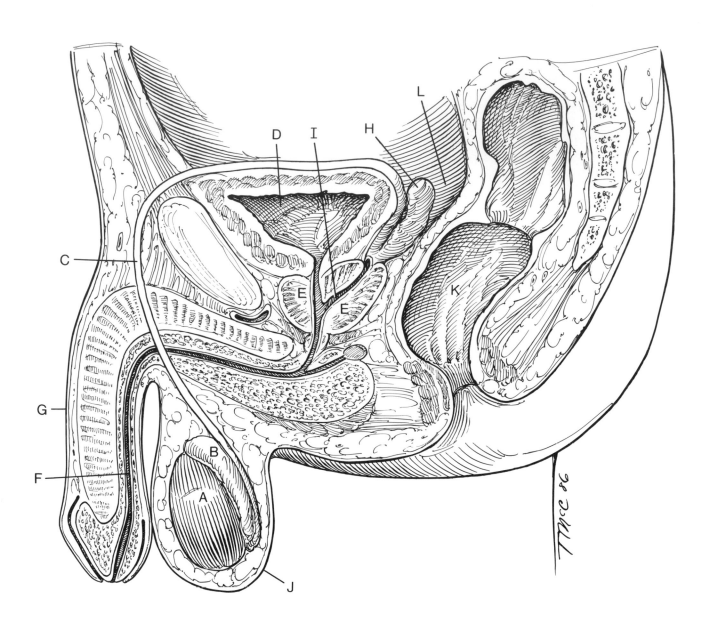

Fig. 8.9  Male Pelvis:  Mid-sagittal View

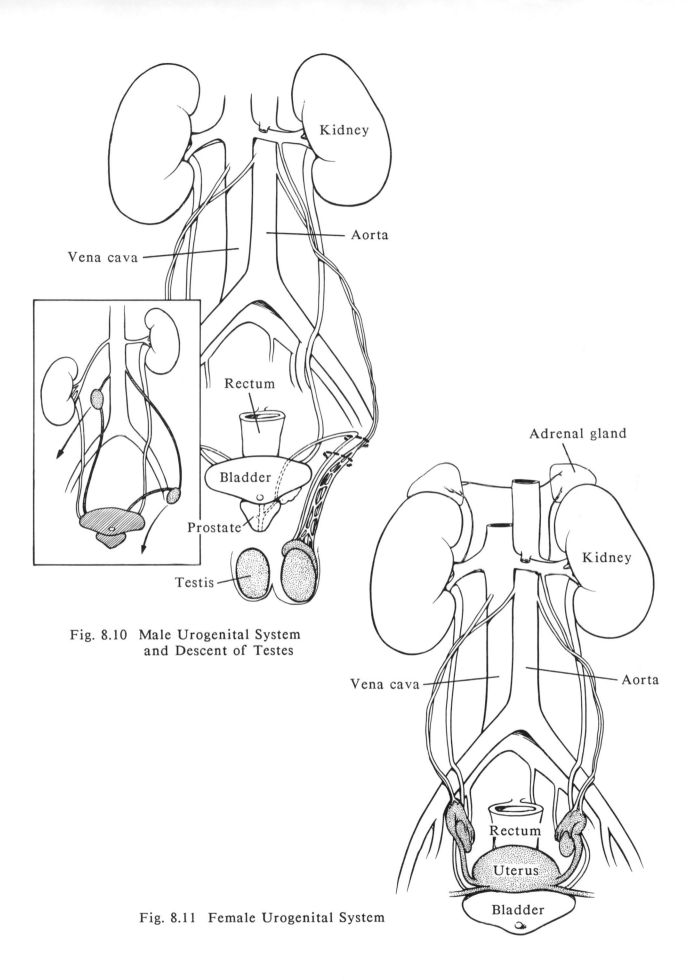

Fig. 8.10  Male Urogenital System
and Descent of Testes

Fig. 8.11  Female Urogenital System

91

What layers of the abdominal wall would the testes pass through on their way o the scrotum, and in what order?

_____

_____

_____

_____

On the inner aspect of the abdominal wall you will find the deep inguinal ring. At this point the vas deferens joins with the other structures mentioned above to pass through the abdominal wall. The pathway through the wall is the inguinal canal. In what layer of the abdominal wall is the deep inguinal ring found? _____ _____ In what layer of the abdominal wall is the superficial ring found? _____
(Refer to Figures 8.1 and 8.2.)


## FOR REVIEW AND THOUGHT

You should be able to trace spermatozoa from their site of production through the genital structures to their site of ejaculation, naming all accessory sex structures along their course.

Similarly, you should be familiar with the female reproductive organs. What is the most common position of the uterus? What is meant by a tubal pregnancy? Where are the fornices of the vagina and what is their significance?

Describe the venous drainage through the hepatic portal system. What is the rationale of such a system? What organs are drained by it? Are any connections with the systemic venous drainage possible?

Be able to assign at least one important function to each organ you have studied in this exercise!

Study Figures 8.12 and 8.13 and note the differences in male and female pelvic skeletal structure.

Use Figures 8.14 - 8.17 and the outline that follows to review the vascular supply of the thorax, abdomen, and pelvis.

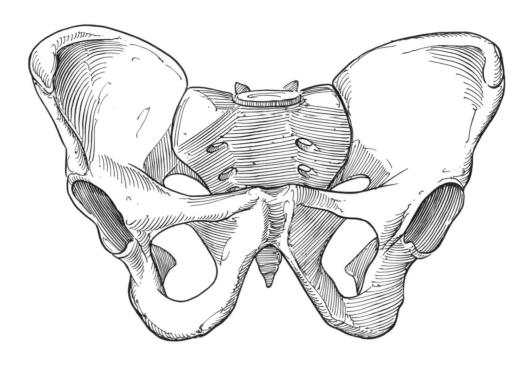

Fig. 8.12 Male Pelvis

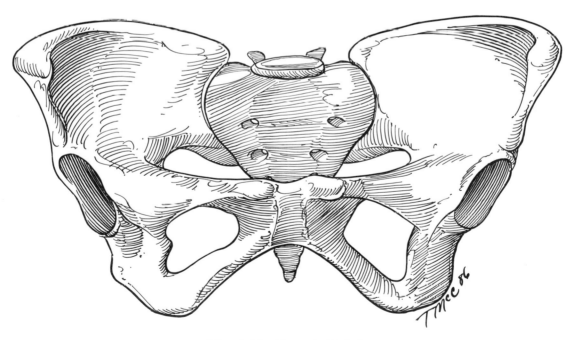

Fig. 8.13 Female Pelvis

93

## CIRCULATORY SYSTEM OUTLINE

## THORAX, ABDOMEN, PELVIS

## <u>ARTERIAL</u>

**Descending Aorta** - A continuation of the ascending aorta and aortic arch; begins at the lower border of the 4th thoracic vertebra and ends at the bifurcation of the aorta anterior to L4 vertebra.

I. **Thoracic Aorta** - from lower border of T4 to the diaphragm (Figure 8.14)

    A.   **Bronchial**

    B.   **Esophageal branches**

    C.   **Pericardial branches**

    D.   **Mediastinal branches**

    E.   **Posterior intercostal** - nine pair usually; supply intercostal spaces 3-11*

    F.   **Subcostal** - inferior to rib 12 (not pictured)

    G.   **Superior phrenic** - to posterior superior surface of the diaphragm

*Anterior intercostal arteries are branches from the internal thoracic artery and one of its terminal branches, the musculophrenic. In addition, the two superiormost intercostal spaces are supplied by the supreme thoracic artery, a branch of the axillary.

II. **Abdominal Aorta** - from the diaphragm to the bifurcation at L4 level. Several schemes exist for describing the branches of the abdominal aorta. In the present outline the branches will be grouped by function rather than in sequential order or origin from the aorta (which is variable from one subject to another) (Figures 8.15 and 8.16).

Numbers 1-3 represent unpaired visceral branches supplying structures that developed from embryonic fore-, mid-, and hindgut respectively.

    H.   **Celiac trunk**

        1.   Left gastric - lesser curve of stomach from left to right

        2.   Common hepatic - to liver

            a.   Gastroduodenal

                (1)   Superior pancreatico-duodenal

                (2)   Right gastroepiploic - greater curve of stomach from right to left

        b.     Right gastric - lesser curve of stomach from right to left

        c.     Proper hepatic - continuation of common hepatic to liver

            (3)   Cystic - gallbladder

3.    Splenic - spleen; pancreas

        d.     Left gastroepiploic - greater curve of stomach from left to right

I.   **Superior mesenteric** - arises from the aorta a short distance inferior to the celiac trunk; supplies part of the duodenum, all of the small intestine, cecum, appendix, ascending colon, and the proximal half of the transverse colon.

4.    Inferior pancreatico-duodenal

5.    Jejunal branches

6.    Ileal branches

7.    Ileocolic

        a.     Appendicular - appendix

8.    Right colic - ascending colon

9.    Middle colic - transverse colon

J.   **Inferior mesenteric** - arises from the aorta behind, or just distal to, the duodenum; supplies the distal half of the transverse colon, descending, and sigmoid colon.

10.   Left colic - half of transverse colon and descending colon

11.   Sigmoid - sigmoid colon

12.   Superior rectal (hemorrhoidal) - continuation of the inferior mesenteric into the pelvis, supplies superior portion of rectum

Letters K-M represent paired branches to glands.

K.   **Suprarenal** - to adrenal glands

L.   **Renal** - to kidneys

M. **Gonadal** - generally arise superior to the origin of the inferior mesenteric

ovarian - female

testicular - male

Letters N-P represent branches to body wall structures.

N. **Inferior phrenic** - inferior surface of diaphragm

O. **Lumbar** - usually four pair, to muscles and skin of back; psoas major, and quadratus lumborum

P. **Median sacral** - direct continuation of the aorta; courses on the ventral surface of the sacrum

**Bifurcation of the Aorta** - The aorta bifurcates into the common iliac arteries at the level of the body of the fourth lumbar vertebra. The common iliacs form internal and external iliac arteries at the level of the fifth lumbar vertebra. The internal iliacs pass into the pelvis to supply muscles and viscera, while the external iliacs continue into the lower limb.

## III. Internal Iliac

Q. **Iliolumbar** - psoas major; quadratus lumborum; ilium

R. **Lateral sacral**

S. **Obturator** - pelvic muscles; hip joint ; anterior and medial thigh

T. **Internal pudendal** - external genitalia

U. **Superior gluteal**

V. **Inferior gluteal**

W. **Umbilical** - a remnant; only partially patent

X. **Visceral branches to the urinary bladder, rectum, prostate, uterus, and vagina**

## IV. External Iliac

Y. **Inferior epigastric** - abdominal wall; peritoneum; cremaster muscle

Z. **Deep iliac circumflex**

## V. Internal Thoracic

This artery contributes significantly to the arterial supply of the thorax and abdomen (Figure 8.14). Label the following branches of this artery.

1. Anterior intercostal - intercostal spaces 1 through 6

2. Musculophrenic - intercostal spaces 7 and below; abdominal muscles

3. Superior epigastric - the terminal continuation of the internal thoracic; abdominal muscles

## VENOUS

I. **Visceral veins do not drain directly into the inferior vena cava, but instead pass through the hepatic portal system (Figure 8.17).**

The inferior mesenteric vein drains into the splenic vein which, in turn, joins the superior mesenteric vein to form the portal vein. The portal vein passes into the liver, breaks up into a network of sinusoidal capillaries, and exits the superior surface of the liver as the hepatic veins (usually two), which enter the inferior vena cava just prior to its passage through the diaphragm. Notice that the hepatic portal system includes the venous drainage of the viscera served by the celiac trunk and the superior and inferior mesenteric arteries.

A. **Inferior mesenteric**

B. **Splenic**

C. **Superior mesenteric**

D. **Portal**

E. **Hepatic sinusoids**

F. **Hepatic veins**

G. **Inferior vena cava**

II. **The systemic veins of the abdomen and pelvis generally accompany the arteries and are given the same names. They drain into the inferior vena cava, which is formed at the level of L4 by the union of the two common iliac veins, each of which, in turn, has received drainage from the internal and external iliac veins.**

The veins commonly draining into the inferior vena cava are:

A. **Lumbar** - usually four pair

B. **Gonadal** - right side only; the left gonadal vein empties into the left renal vein

C. **Renal**

D. **Suprarenal** - usually right side only; left empties into the renal vein

E.    **Inferior phrenic**

F.    **Hepatic**

III.   **Systemic Veins of the Thorax (not pictured)**

G.    **Internal thoracic** - paired; drain into the brachiocephalic veins

1.    Superior epigastric

2.    Musculophrenic

3.    Anterior intercostal

H.    **Azygos and Hemiazygos veins** - azygos on right, hemiazygos on left; drain the posterior thoracic wall; the posterior intercostal veins are the main contributors to this drainage.  The hemiazygos crosses the anterior surface of the vertebral column to join the azygos, which then empties into the superior vena cava just prior to its entrance into the right atrium.

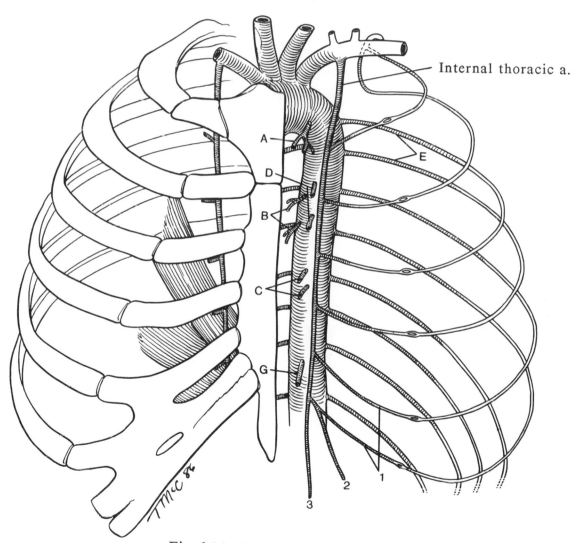

Internal thoracic a.

Fig. 8.14  Thoracic Arteries

99

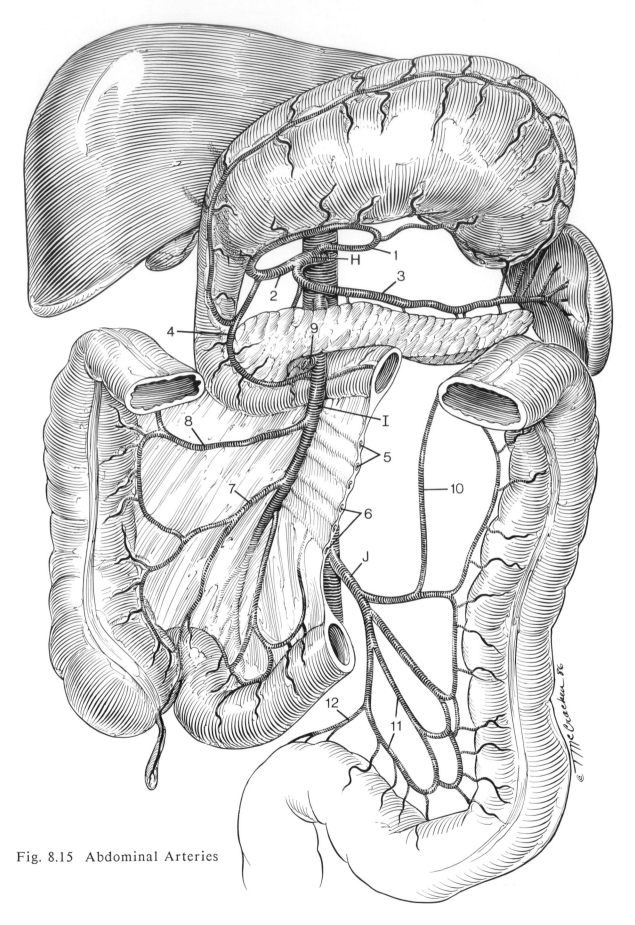

Fig. 8.15  Abdominal Arteries

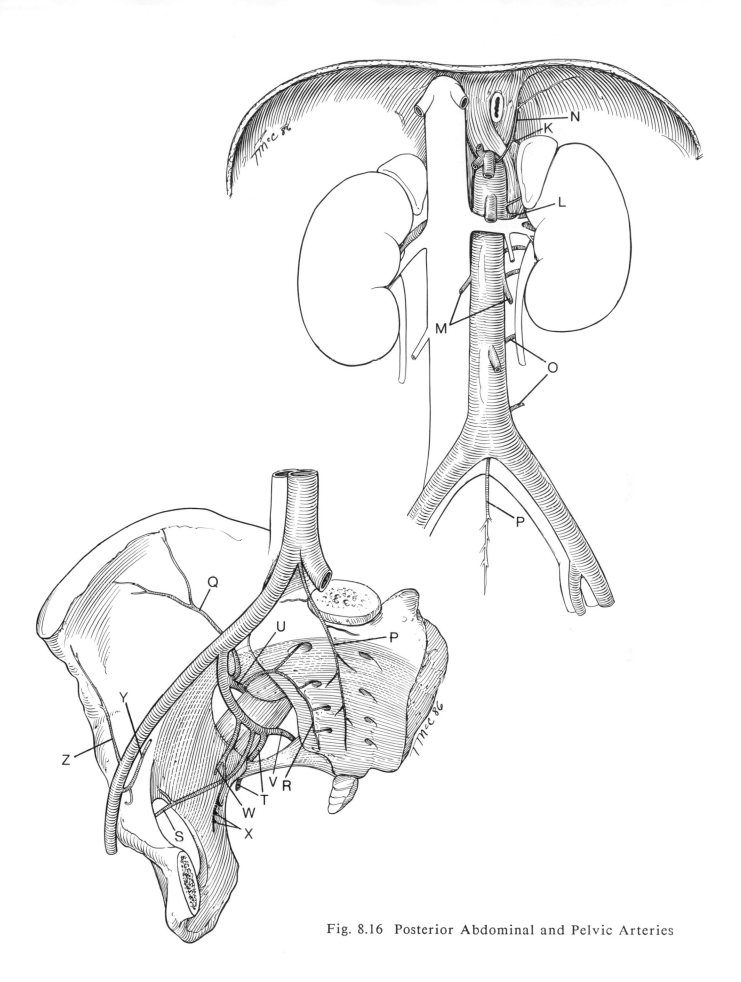

Fig. 8.16  Posterior Abdominal and Pelvic Arteries

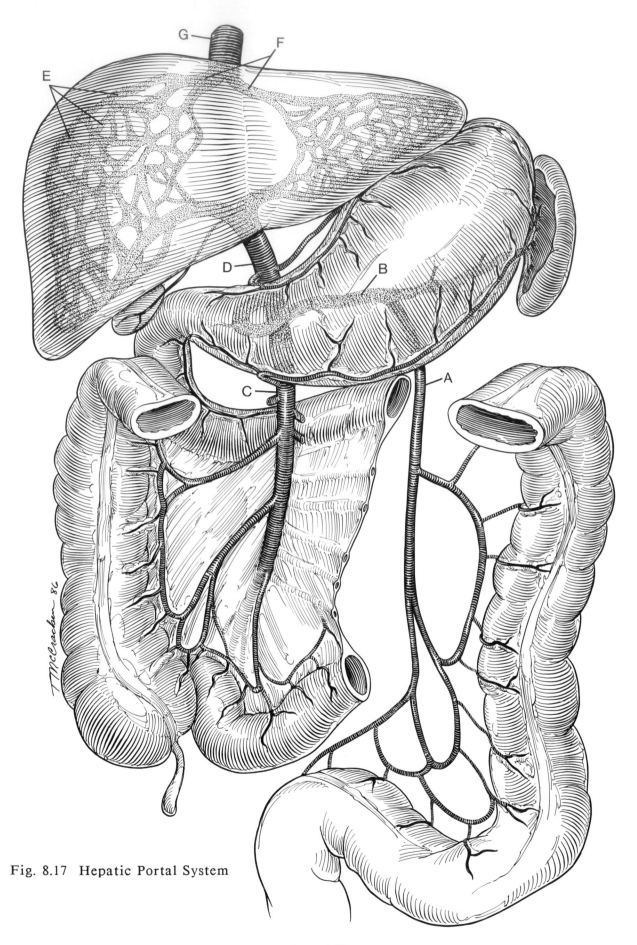

Fig. 8.17  Hepatic Portal System

## EXERCISE 9.  BONES OF THE SKULL

This exercise provides you with an introduction to the bones of the face and cranium.  If possible, use skulls to find the bones and features described and label the figures in this exercise properly.  The terminology presented will be encountered throughout your study of the head and neck, so begin to acquaint yourself with it now.

I.   **Bones of the Cranium (Figures 9.1 and 9.2) - These bones are mainly for protection of cranial contents; some are singular and some paired.**

    A.    **Frontal**

    B.    **Occipital**

    C.    **Sphenoid**

    D.    **Ethmoid**

    E.    **Temporal (2)**

    F.    **Parietal (2)**

II.   **Bones of the Face (Figures 9.1 and 9.2)**

    G.    **Mandible**

    H.    **Vomer (Figure 9.4)**

    I.    **Maxillary (2)**

    J.    **Zygomatic (2)**

    K.    **Nasal (2)**

    L.    **Lacrimal (2)**

    M.    **Palatine (2) (Figure 9.4)**

    N.    **Inferior nasal conchae (2)**

III.   **Organization, Foramina, Landmarks**

With the cranial cap (calvarium) removed and looking into the cranial cavity, one notices three step-like fossae.  These are the anterior, middle, and posterior cranial fossae.  We will utilize these fossae in studying the internal features of the cranium (Figure 9.3).

    A.    **Anterior cranial fossa** - This fossa lies superior to the orbits and houses the frontal lobes of the brain.  Find the following in this fossa:

        1.    Frontal bone

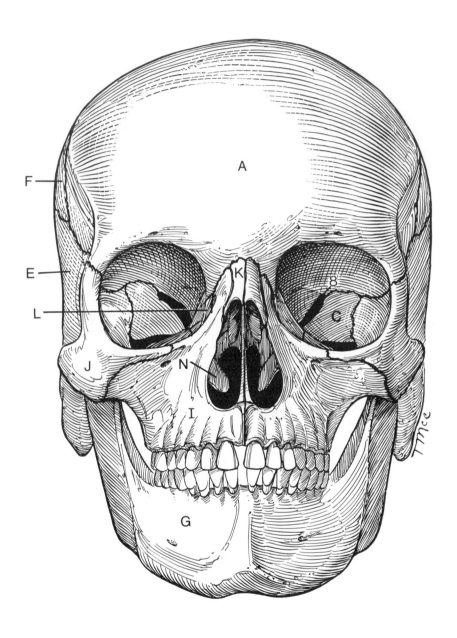

Fig. 9.1 Anterior View of Skull

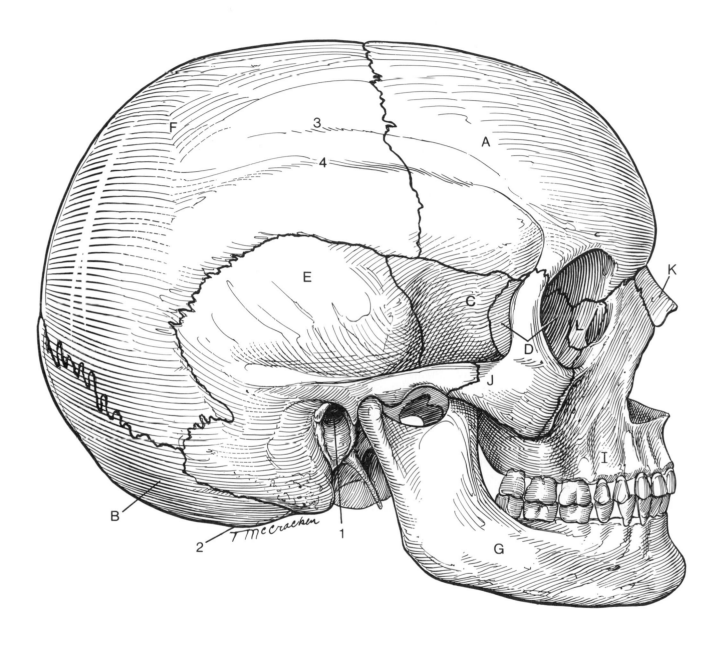

Fig. 9.2  Lateral View of Skull

2. Cribriform plates

3. Crista galli

B. **Middle cranial fossa** - The middle cranial fossa houses the temporal lobes of the brain and lies posterior to the orbits. Find the following in this fossa:

**Sphenoid bone**

4. Lesser wing

5. Greater wing

6. Sella turcica

7. Optic foramen

8. Superior orbital fissure (Figure 9.1 also)

9. Foramen rotundum

10. Foramen ovale

11. Foramen spinosum

**Temporal bone**

12. Carotid canal

13. Foramen lacerum

14. Squamous portion with groove for the middle meningeal artery

15. Petrous portion with grooves for the superior and inferior petrosal sinuses

C. **Posterior cranial fossa** - This is the largest and deepest of the three fossae and houses the cerebellum and medulla. Find the following in this fossa:

**Temporal bone**

16. Internal auditory meatus

17. Jugular foramen

**Occipital bone**

18. Hypoglossal canal

19. Basilar portion

20. Foramen magnum

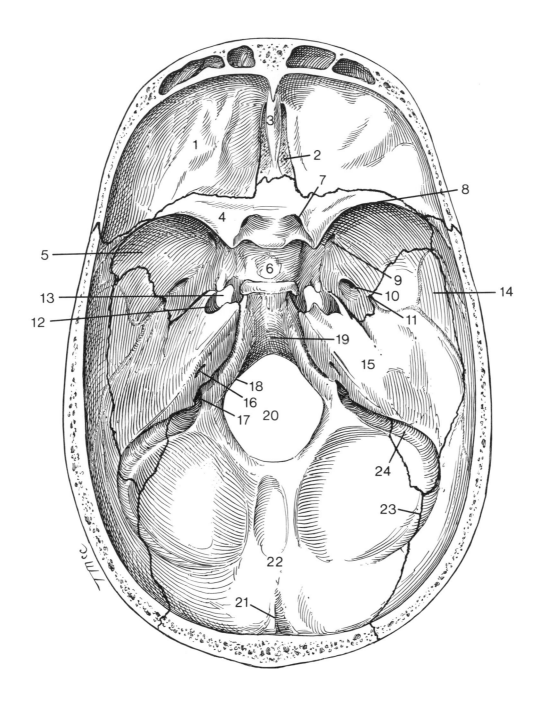

Fig. 9.3 Interior View of Skull

107

21. Internal occipital crest

22. Groove for the confluence of sinus

23. Groove for transverse sinus

24. Groove for sigmoid sinus

D. **Base of skull (Figure 9.4)** - Find the following on the inferior aspect of the skull.

1. Hard palate

2. Mandibular fossa

3. Mastoid process

4. Styloid process

5. Stylomastoid foramen

6. Pterygoid plates (medial and lateral)

7. Sphenoid spine

8. Carotid canal

9. Occipital condyle

10. Foramen magnum

11. External occipital protuberance

12. Superior nuchal line

13. Inferior nuchal line

E. **Superficial features of the face and cranium (Figure 9.2)**

1. External auditory meatus

2. External occipital protuberance

3. Superior temporal line

4. Inferior temporal line

F. **Mandible (Figures 9.5 and 9.6)**

1. Body

2. Ramus

3. Angle

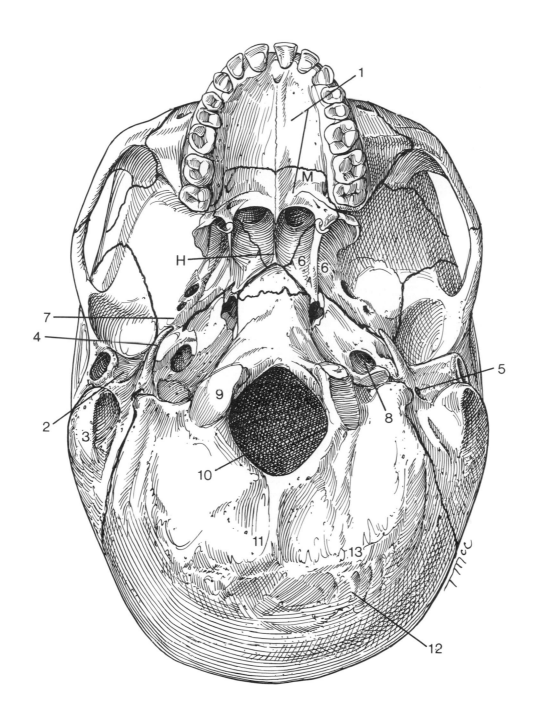

Fig. 9.4  Base of Skull

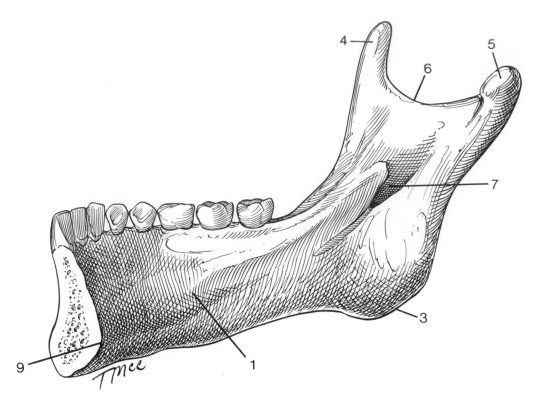

Fig. 9.5  Medial View Mandible

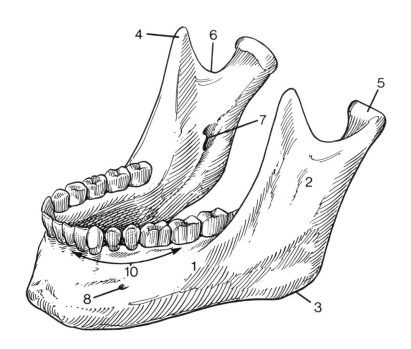

Fig. 9.6  3/4 View Mandible

4. Coronoid process

5. Condyloid process, with condyle

6. Mandibular notch

7. Mandibular foramen

8. Mental foramen

9. Genial tubercle

10. Alveolar process

## FOR REVIEW AND THOUGHT

Find the orbital cavity and identify the bones contributing to the boundaries of this cavity.

**Roof =**

**Floor =**

**Lateral wall =**

**Medial wall =**

Find the hard palate and list the bones involved in forming this structure.

On the face find the supra and infraorbital foramina (the supraorbital is often a notch rather than a foramen). Notice that these two foramina fall in a perpendicular line with the mental foramen on the mandible. This will be of significance during study of the cranial nerves because a branch of each division of the trigeminal nerve exits each of these foramina.

# EXERCISE 10. NECK AND FACE

The purpose of this exercise is the identification, study, and appreciation of important structures in the neck and face. The neck is a key region because of the passage of many structures through it. This concept of the continuity of structures from head to thorax (or vice versa) through the neck is very important to your understanding of this area.

I.  **Neck (Figures 10.1 and 10.2)**

The neck is geographically divided into triangles (Figure 10.1) each with specific boundaries. The two main divisions are the anterior and posterior triangles. The anterior triangle is bounded by the cervical midline medially, the sternocleidomastoid muscle laterally, and the body of the mandible superiorly. The subdivisions of the anterior triangle are as follows:

A.  **Submandibular** - bounded by the bellies of the digastric muscle posteriorly and anteriorly and by the body of the mandible superiorly.

B.  **Carotid** - bounded by the sternocleidomastoid posteriorly, the superior belly of the omohyoid muscle anteriorly, and the posterior belly of the digastric superiorly.

C.  **Muscular** - bounded by the cervical midline medially, by the superior belly of the omohyoid superolaterally, and by the sternocleidomastoid inferolaterally.

D.  **Submental** - bounded medially by the cervical midline, by the anterior belly of the digastric laterally, and by the hyoid bone inferiorly.

The posterior triangle is bounded by the trapezius posteriorly, the sterno-cleidomastoid anteriorly, and the clavicle inferiorly. The posterior triangle is subdivided as follows:

E.  **Occipital** - bounded anteriorly and posteriorly as described above and inferiorly by the posterior belly of the omohyoid.

F.  **Omoclavicular** - bounded anteriorly by the sternocleidomastoid, superiorly by the posterior belly of the omohyoid, and inferiorly by the clavicle.

**Other neck structures are shown in Figure 10.2.**

A.  **External jugular vein** - found on the superficial surface of the sternocleido-mastoid.

B.  **Sternohyoid** - this is found in the muscular triangle. What are the proximal and distal attachments of this muscle?

PA -

DA -

C.  **Sternothyroid**

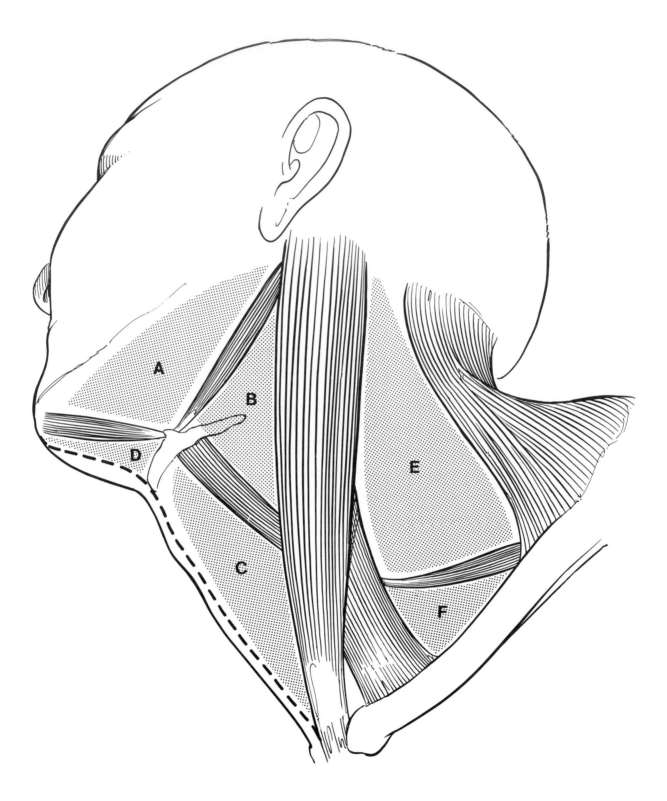

Fig. 10.1  Triangles of Neck

114

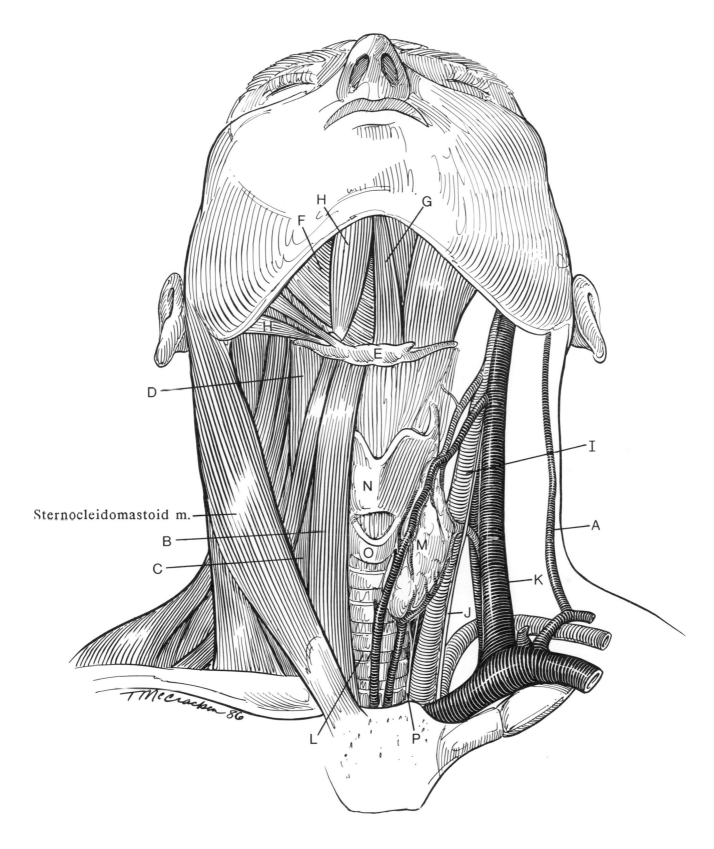

Sternocleidomastoid m.

Fig. 10.2 Anterior Neck

D.  **Thyrohyoid**

These muscles are found deep to the sternohyoid.  The proximal and distal attachments of these muscles should be obvious to you.  Note that all of these muscles are paired (bilateral).  These muscles are, as a group, called the infrahyoid strap muscles.  What, then, would you consider the function of this group of muscles to be?

_____

E.  **Hyoid bone** - Find the hyoid bone in Figure 10.2 and on yourself.  To do this place your thumb and index finger on the angles of your mandible, tip up your chin,  slide your thumb and finger anteriorly about 1 1/2 inches, and press gently.

F.  **Mylohyoid**

G.  **Geniohyoid**

H.  **Digastric (anterior and posterior bellies)**

These are collectively known as suprahyoid muscles.  List the attachments of these muscles below.

**Mylohyoid** -   PA -

DA -

**Geniohyoid** -   PA -

DA -

**Digastric** -    PA -

DA -

What would be the collective function of these muscles?

_____

Find your hyoid bone again and swallow.  What happens to the hyoid bone when you do this?

_____

Lateral and deep to the superior belly of the omohyoid is the carotid sheath. The sheath is a layer of connective tissue enveloping three important structures:

I.  **Common carotid artery**

J.  **Vagus nerve**

K.  **Internal jugular vein**

Other structures to find in the neck include (Figure 10.2):

L. **Trachea**

M. **Thyroid gland**

N. **Thyroid cartilage**

O. **Cricoid cartilage**

P. **Recurrent laryngeal nerve** - In the groove between the trachea and esophagus the recurrent laryngeal nerves ascend to reach the larynx. You learned of these nerves in Exercise 6. From what cranial nerve are these branches?

_____

Describe briefly the course of these nerves and any differences between the right and left sides.

_____

_____

II. **Face**

Identify the following muscles (Figure 10.3).

A. **Platysma**

B. **Orbicularis oculi**

C. **Orbicularis oris**

D. **Zygomaticus**

E. **Masseter**

F. **Buccinator** (deep and anterior to the masseter)

Posterior to the masseter find the following structures.

G. **Parotid gland**

H. **Parotid duct** - passes from the gland over the superficial surface of the masseter and pierces the buccinator to empty into the oral cavity

I. **Facial** (VII cranial) nerve - This nerve appears to emerge from the parotid gland. In reality it passes through a fine fascial septum in the gland and emerges on the face to split into five main branches. List the five branches.

_____

_____

_____

_____

_____

The facial nerve branches seen here are motor nerves to the muscles of facial expression.

Three superficial branches of the trigeminal (V cranial) nerve can be found on the face.

The supraorbital nerve emerges from the supraorbital notch or foramen. This nerve is a branch of the ophthalmic division of the trigeminal nerve (V1).

The infraorbital nerve emerges from the infraorbital foramen. This nerve is a branch of the maxillary division of the trigeminal nerve (V2).

The third superficial nerve is a branch of the mandibular division of the trigeminal nerve (V3). It is the mental nerve and is found exiting the mental foramen.

The area of sensory distribution of the three divisions of the trigeminal nerve is shown in Figure 10.4.

## FOR REVIEW AND THOUGHT

The first portion of this exercise dealt with the triangles of the neck and their boundaries. Now that you have studied the neck and face list the important contents of the various triangles.

Figure 10.5 provides a conceptual look at the twelve cranial nerves. Using this illustration and any supplemental information you have learned, begin to fill in the table on the following pages.

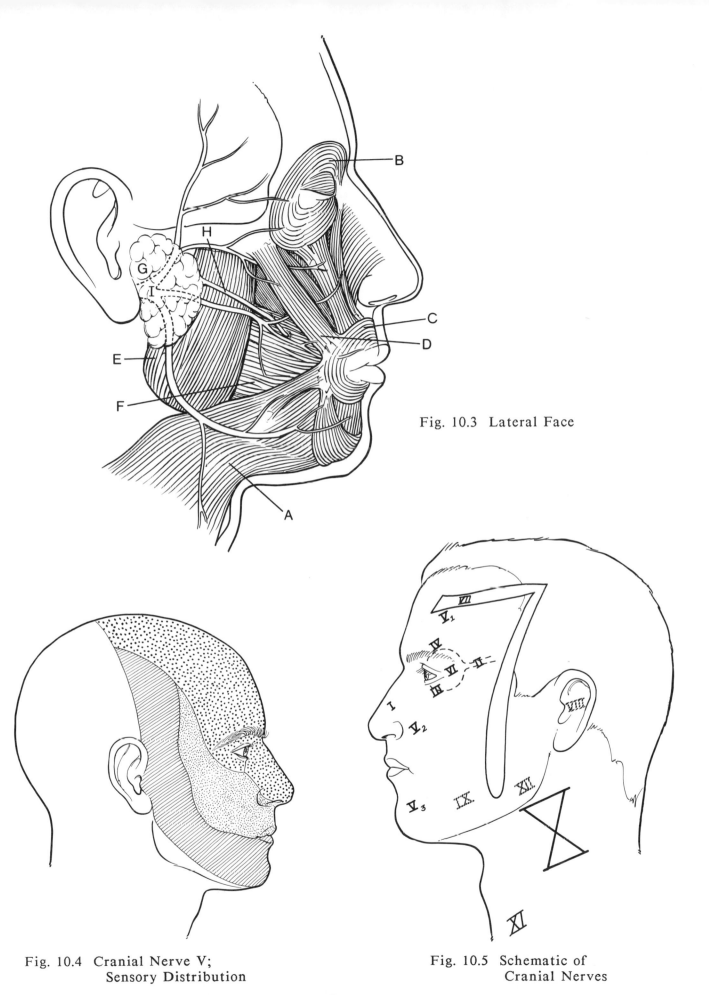

Fig. 10.3 Lateral Face

Fig. 10.4 Cranial Nerve V;
Sensory Distribution

Fig. 10.5 Schematic of
Cranial Nerves

119

CRANIAL NERVES

| NAME | MOTOR | SENSORY | SPECIAL SENSORY | AUTONOMIC | FORAMEN OF EXIT |
|------|-------|---------|-----------------|-----------|-----------------|
| I | | | | | |
| II | | | | | |
| III | | | | | |
| IV | | | | | |
| V $V_1$ | | | | | |
| V $V_2$ | | | | | |
| V $V_3$ | | | | | |

CRANIAL NERVES (continued)

| NAME | MOTOR | SENSORY | SPECIAL SENSORY | AUTONOMIC | FORAMEN OF EXIT |
|------|-------|---------|-----------------|-----------|-----------------|
| VI | | | | | |
| VII | | | | | |
| VIII | | | | | |
| IX | | | | | |
| X | | | | | |
| XI | | | | | |
| XII | | | | | |

121

# NOTES

# EXERCISE 11. BRAIN AND ORGANS OF SPEECH, VISION, AND HEARING

## I. Bisected Head

Figure 11.1 illustrates a slightly parasagittal section of the head and neck. Observe and label the following structures.

A. **Cerebral hemisphere with gyri and sulci**

B. **Corpus callosum**

C. **Interventricular foramen** (of Munro)

D. **Pituitary gland in sella turcica**

E. **Third ventricle**

F. **Thalamus**

G. **Hypothalamus**

H. **Cerebral aqueduct** (of Sylvius)

I. **Midbrain**

J. **Fourth ventricle**

K. **Pons**

L. **Cerebellum**

M. **Choroid plexus** (tufts of vascular tissue within the ventricles)

N. **Medulla**

O. **Nasal cavity**

P. **Nasal conchae**

Q. **Oral cavity**

R. **Soft palate**

S. **Epiglottis**

T. **Frontal sinus**

U. **Sphenoid sinus**

V. **Vestibular fold of larynx**

W. **Vocal fold of larynx**

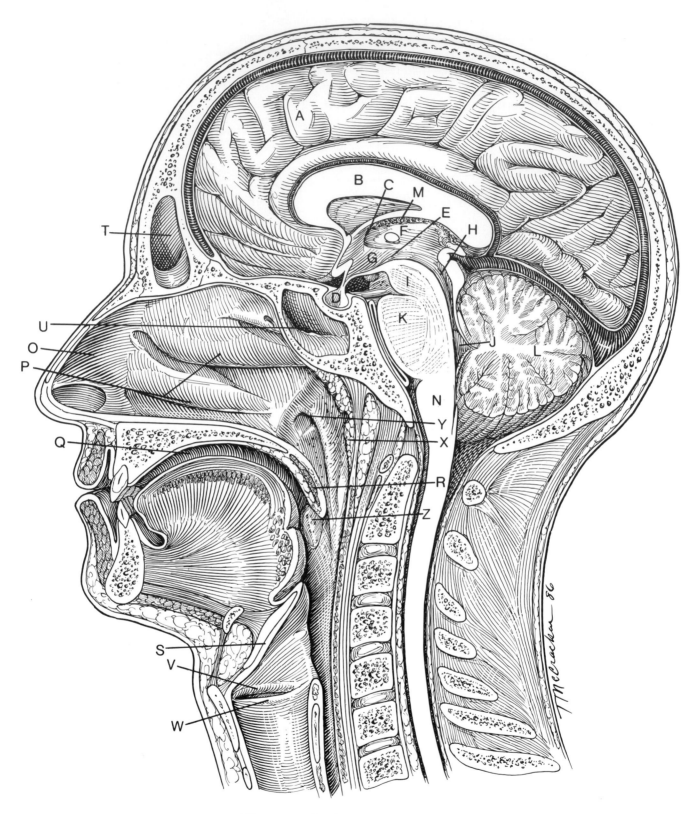

Fig. 11.1  Sagittal Section, Head

## II. Dural Folds

The dura mater surrounding the spinal cord is continuous with that surrounding the brain, the other portion of the central nervous system. In the cranium this dura mater is thrown into folds separating the cerebral and cerebellar hemispheres sagittally and the cerebellum from the cerebrum transversely (Figure 11.2). Venous drainage of the brain is accomplished through channels in these dural folds, known as venous sinuses.

These folds are the falx cerebri, falx cerebelli, and tentorium cerebelli. Beside these below, write the portions of the brain they separate.

A. **Falx cerebri**

B. **Falx cerebelli**

C. **Tentorium cerebelli**

Using Figures 11.2 and 11.3, find the following venous sinuses.

D. **Superior sagittal**

E. **Inferior sagittal**

F. **Confluence**

G. **Straight**

H. **Transverse**

I. **Sigmoid**

Next to each of these sinuses, write the dural fold in which they are found.

The sigmoid sinus forms the internal jugular vein at the jugular foramen.

## III. Pharynx and Larynx

The pharynx lies anterior to the vertebral column and is subdivided into nasal, oral, and laryngeal portions (Figure 11.1).

### Nasopharynx

The nasopharynx is located at the posterior end of the nasal cavity and superior to the soft palate. Two important structures are found in the nasopharynx. Label these on Figure 11.1.

X. **Pharyngeal tonsil**

Y. **Opening of the auditory (pharyngotympanic, eustachian) tube**

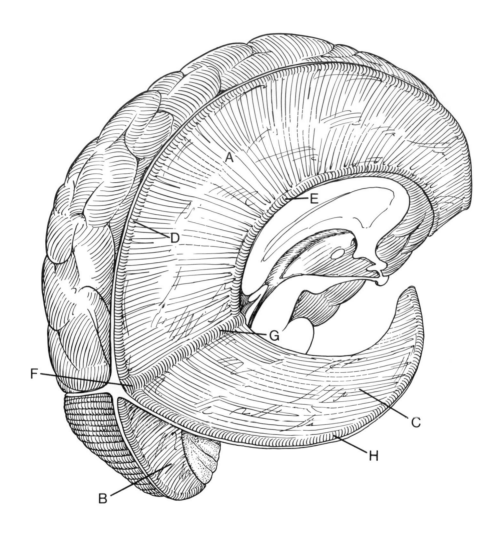

Fig. 11.2  Dural Folds and Venous Sinuses

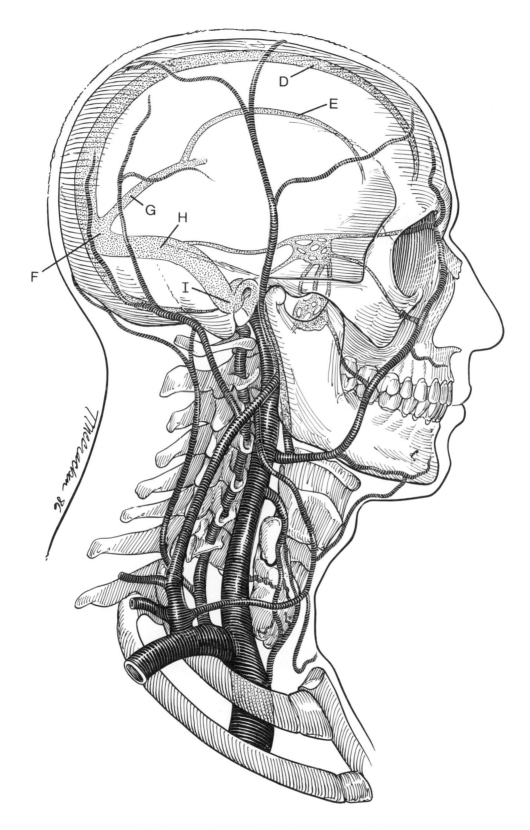

Fig. 11.3  Venous Drainage of Head

## Oropharynx

The oropharynx is located at the posterior end of the oral cavity, inferior to the soft palate, and superior to the opening of the larynx. Find the palatine tonsils in the oropharynx!

Z.   **Palatine tonsil**

## Laryngopharynx

The laryngopharynx contains the larynx. The laryngopharynx is continued inferiorly as the esophagus posteriorly and the trachea anteriorly. The larynx consists of a cartilagenous skeleton with associated muscles and mucous membranes. The cartilages of the larynx include:

A.   **Thyroid**

B.   **Epiglottic**

C.   **Cricoid**

D.   **Arytenoid**

E.   **Corniculate**

Of these, the paired arytenoids, the cricoid, and the thyroid are crucial in phonation. Label A through E above in Figure 11.4.

Just anterior to the vertebral column is a layer of prevertebral fascia, and anterior to this fascia are the pharyngeal constrictor muscles. The pharyngeal constrictors are three in number (superior, middle, inferior) and form the posterior boundary of the pharynx (Figure 11.4).

F.   **Superior**

G.   **Middle**

H.   **Inferior**

Several muscles are important in regulating phonation and inspiration/expiration by acting upon the cartilages of the larynx to abduct, adduct, or tense the vocal cords. Next to each of the muscles listed, write their action and innervation.

I.   **Cricothyroid**

J.   **Posterior cricoarytenoid**

K.   **Lateral cricoarytenoid**

L.   **Transverse arytenoid**

M.   **Oblique arytenoid**

128

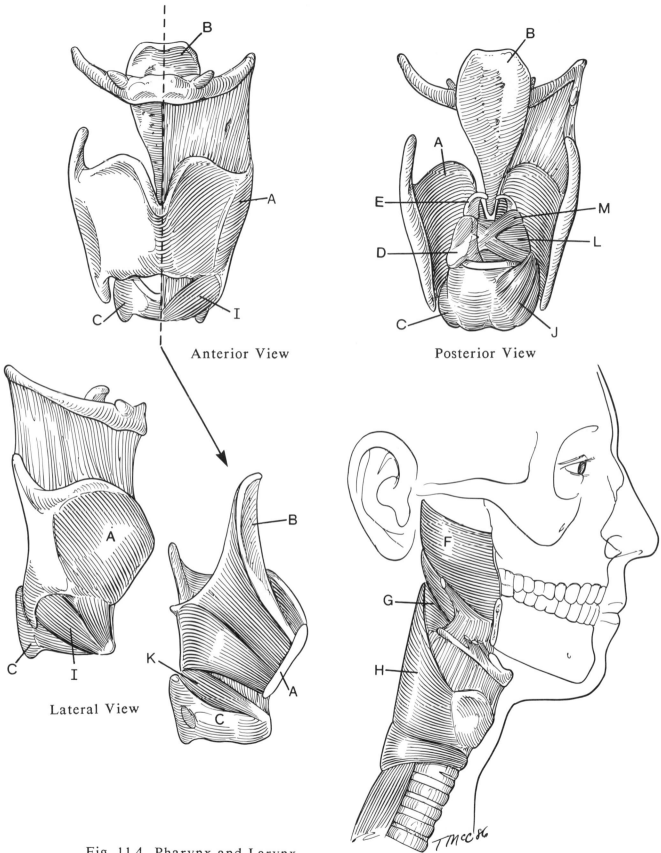

Anterior View

Posterior View

Lateral View

Fig. 11.4 Pharynx and Larynx

129

Figures 11.5 and 11.6 provide sagittal and superior views of the orbit. Identify the following in these figures.

A.   **Optic nerve**

B.   **Fibrous layer** - sclera, with its anterior extension, the cornea ($B_1$)

C.   **Vascular layer** - choroid (C); ciliary body ($C_2$); iris ($C_3$)

D.   **Nervous layer** - retina

E.   **Anterior and posterior chambers** - both filled with aqueous humor

F.   **Vitreous body**

G.   **Lens**

H.   **Suspensory ligaments**

I.   **Orbicularis oculi**

J.   **Superior and inferior palpebrae with tarsal plates**

K.   **Levator palpebrae superioris**

L.   **Superior rectus**

M.   **Conjoined fascia of levator palpebrae superioris and superior rectus**

N.   **Inferior rectus**

O.   **Lateral rectus**

P.   **Medial rectus**

Q.   **Superior oblique**

R.   **Trochlea**

S.   **Inferior oblique**

Figure 11.7 shows the ear. Label the following structures.

A.   **External ear**

   1.   Auricle or pinna

   2.   External auditory meatus and canal

   3.   Tympanic membrane

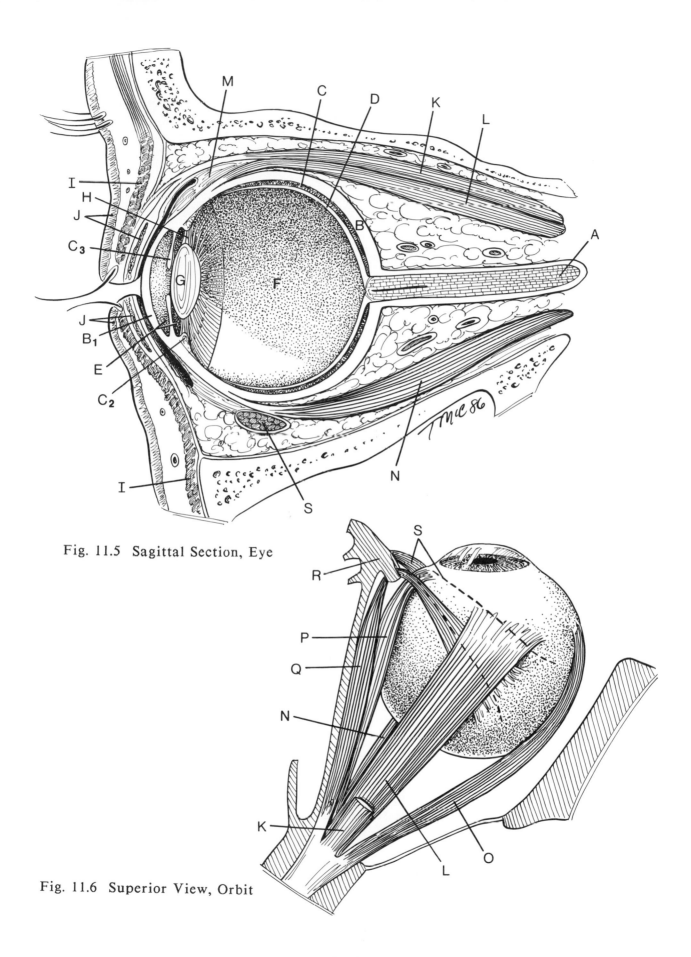

Fig. 11.5  Sagittal Section, Eye

Fig. 11.6  Superior View, Orbit

B. **Middle ear**

    4. Tympanic cavity

    5. Malleus

    6. Incus

    7. Stapes

    8. Auditory tube

    9. Oval window

    10. Round window

    11. Chorda tympani

C. **Inner ear**

    12. Semicircular canals

    13. Cochlea

    14. Vestibular portion of vestibulocochlear nerve (VIII cranial)

    15. Cochlear portion of vestibulocochlear nerve (VIII cranial)

## FOR REVIEW AND THOUGHT

List the six extraocular muscles with their actions on the eyeball and their innervations.

With your study partners discuss these questions:

What is the anatomical reason for the association of middle ear infections with sore throats, colds, and inflammation of the pharyngeal tonsils, especially in young children?

What is infection and swelling of the pharyngeal tonsils called?

What is the nerve supply to the pharynx and larynx? What specific nerves supply the laryngeal muscles?

When you have answered these questions, fill in the remainder of the cranial nerve table you began in Exercise 10.

Use Figures 11.8 - 11.10 and the following outline to review the vascular structures of the head and neck.

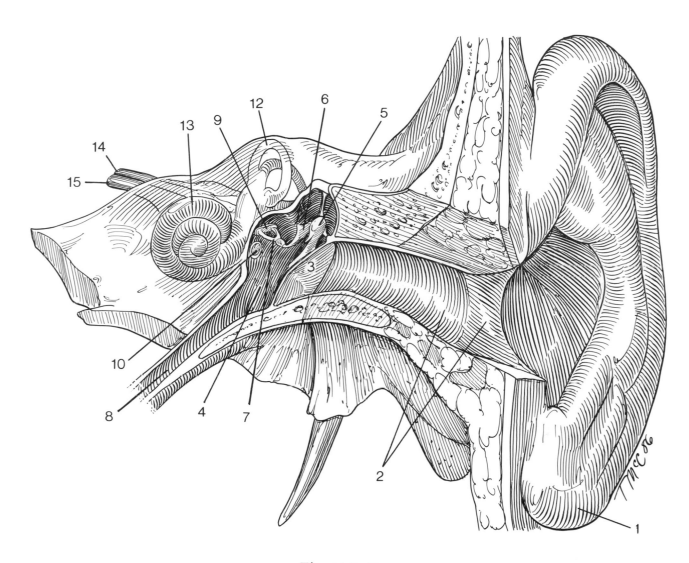

Fig. 11.7  Ear

133

## Aortic Arch

The origin of vessels off the aortic arch is different on the right and left sides. On the right side a brachiocephalic trunk arises, which then divides into the subclavian artery to the upper limb (brachium) and the common carotid artery to the neck and head (cephalo). On the left side these vessels arise separately from the aortic arch. Starting with the common carotids, the arterial supply is "the same" on each side.

## Common Carotid (Figures 11.8 and 11.9)

The common carotid artery has no branches. It bifurcates at approximately the superior border of the thyroid cartilage into external and internal branches. The carotid sinus and carotid body are located at this bifurcation.

### I. External Carotid

Ascends to supply the exterior of the neck, face, and head. Eight major branches are usually described.

A. **Superior thyroid** - thyroid gland

    1. Superior laryngeal

B. **Ascending pharyngeal** - pharynx, palate, tonsil, auditory tube

C. **Lingual** - tongue; also sends branches to the tonsils, soft palate, and suprahyoid muscles

D. **Facial** - muscles and skin of face

    2. Inferior labial - lower lip

    3. Superior labial - upper lip

    4. Angular - terminal continuation of the facial: to the medial angle of the eye

E. **Occipital** - posterior scalp, sternocleidomastoid, trapezius

F. **Posterior auricular** - external ear and part of tympanic membrane

G. **Maxillary** - both jaws, nasal cavity, oral cavity, tympanic membrane, dura mater, lacrimal gland, eye muscles, etc.

    5. Inferior alveolar - mandible and lower teeth

    6. Middle meningeal - dura mater

7.   Buccal - cheek and gums (gingiva)

8.   Infraorbital - upper jaw and teeth

9.   Sphenopalatine - nasal cavity

### H.   Superficial temporal

The maxillary and superficial temporal arteries are considered the terminal branches of the external carotid artery.

## II.   Internal Carotid

The internal carotid artery has no branches in the neck.  It enters the temporal bone and passes through the carotid canal to reach the middle cranial fossa.  Once inside the cranium it is a major supplier to the brain.  The following branches are usually described (Figure 11.9).

### I.   Ophthalmic - enters the orbit via the optic canal

10.   Central artery of the retina

### J.   Anterior cerebral

11.   Anterior communicating

### K.   Posterior communicating

### L.   Anterior choroidal - internal capsule

### M.   Middle cerebral

The middle cerebral artery is considered the terminal continuation of the internal carotid artery

## III.   Other Arteries of the Neck and Head

### Vertebral (Figures 11.8 and 11.9)

The vertebral arteries offer a second route to the brain.  These vessels are the first and largest branches off the subclavian arteries.  To reach the head these vessels pass through the transverse foramina of the cervical vertebrae.  After emerging from the transverse foramina of the first cervical vertebra (atlas), the arteries pass dorsally and medially around the superior articular facets and enter the skull through the foramen magnum.

### N.   Posterior spinal - posterior surface of spinal cord

### O.   Anterior spinal - anterior surface of spinal cord

### P.   Posterior inferior cerebellar - cerebellum

### Q.   Basilar - formed by the union of the two vertebral arteries

135

12. Anterior inferior cerebellar - cerebellum

13. Labyrinthine - internal ear

14. Pontine - usually several pair; supplies pons

15. Superior cerebellar - cerebellum

16. Posterior cerebral - paired; formed by the bifurcation of the basilar artery

    a.    Posterior communicating

## IV. Thyrocervical Trunk (Figure 11.8)

This trunk, also a branch of the subclavian artery, supplies blood to neck structures.

R.    Inferior thyroid - neck, trachea, esophagus, thyroid gland

    17.    Ascending cervical

S.    Suprascapular

T.    Transverse cervical

## V. Circle of Willis (Figure 11.9)

The Circle of Willis is an anastomosis of internal carotid and vertebral arteries at the base of the brain (surrounding the pituitary gland and sella turcica). This anastomosis is established in the following way: The posterior communicating arteries connect the two posterior cerebral arteries with the internal carotid arteries and the anterior communicating artery connects the two anterior cerebral arteries.

# VENOUS

The veins of the face and head are extensive and, for the most part, have names identical to the arteries. Like the arteries, the veins are organized into external and internal systems. These two systems do communicate in several places (Figure 11.10).

## I. External Jugular Vein

The external jugular receives the greater part of the venous drainage from the exterior surface of the cranium and deep face. It is formed on the superficial surface of the sternocleidomastoid muscle at about the level of the angle of the mandible by the union of a portion of the retromandibular vein and the posterior auricular vein. The external jugular ends by emptying into the subclavian vein.

A. **Posterior auricular**

B. **Posterior ramus of the retromandibular** - the retromandibular is formed by the union of the superficial temporal and maxillary veins

C. **Superficial temporal**

D. **Maxillary**

E. **Anterior jugular** - this vein is variable in occurrence. It typically begins by the union of small veins between the hyoid bone and chin. It descends near the ventral midline of the neck and ends in the external jugular vein close to the subclavian vein.

## II. Internal Jugular Vein

The internal jugular collects blood from the inside of the cranium and some from the face and neck. It is formed at the jugular foramen as a direct continuation of the cranial venous drainage. The vessels course inferiorly in the neck in close company with the common carotid artery and the vagus nerve, deep to the sternocleidomastoid muscle. At the root of the neck they unite with the subclavian veins to form the brachiocephalic veins, which in turn form the superior vena cava.

The veins of the brain are tributaries of the internal jugular but empty first into dural venous sinuses. You learned many of the dural sinuses in **Exercise 10**. Some other important sinuses are:

F. **Cavernous**

G. **Superior petrosal**

H. **Inferior petrosal**

As it descends through the neck the internal jugular vein receives venous blood from the other sources.

I. **Facial**

J. **Anterior ramus of the retromandibular**

137

K.   **Superior thyroid**

III.   **Vertebral Venous Plexus** - lying both within and without the vertebral canal

IV.   **Connections Between Superficial and Deep Venous Drainage.** In studying Figure 11.10 you will see sites at which drainages communicate. The facial vein communicates with the ophthalmic veins in the orbit, and through them with the cavernous sinus. The facial vein also communicates with the pterygoid plexus located posterior to the upper molar teeth in the region of the pterygoid plates of the sphenoid plates of the sphenoid bone. The pterygoid plexus, in turn, also communicates with the cavernous sinus and receives drainage from the middle meningeal vein. These anastomoses are of considerable clinical importance because the veins of the face are valveless. Infection may pass from superficial to deep veins with potentially devastating results, especially if the cavernous sinus is involved.

L.   **Pterygoid plexus**

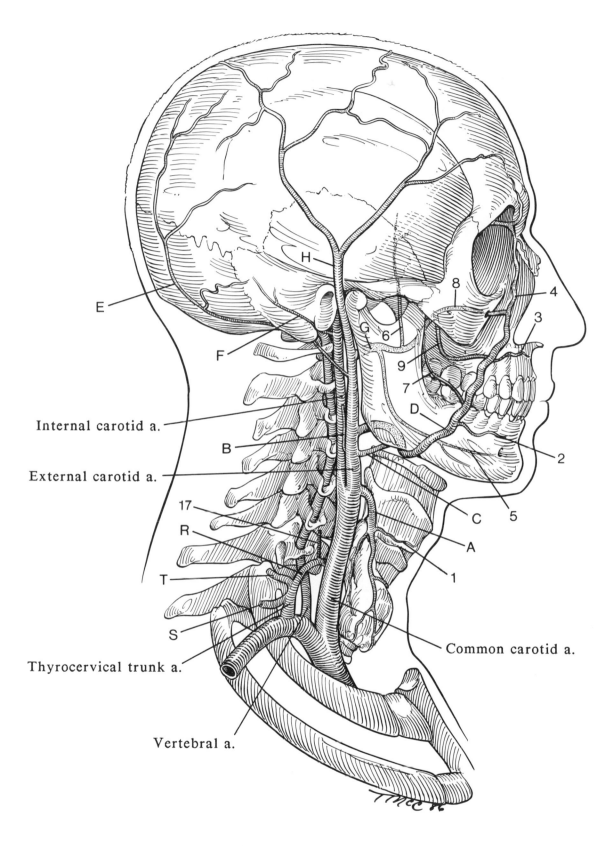

Internal carotid a.

External carotid a.

17

R

T

S

Thyrocervical trunk a.

Vertebral a.

E

F

H

G

6

8

4

3

9

7

D

C

5

2

B

A

1

Common carotid a.

Fig. 11.8    Arterial Supply to Head

139

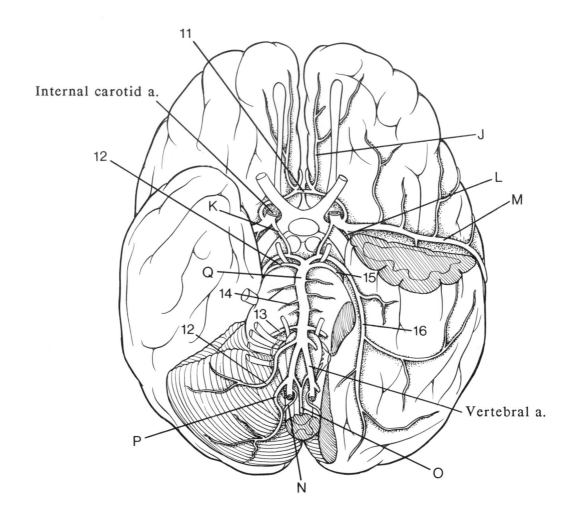

Internal carotid a.

Vertebral a.

Fig. 11.9  Internal Carotid and Vertebral
Arteries and Circle of Willis

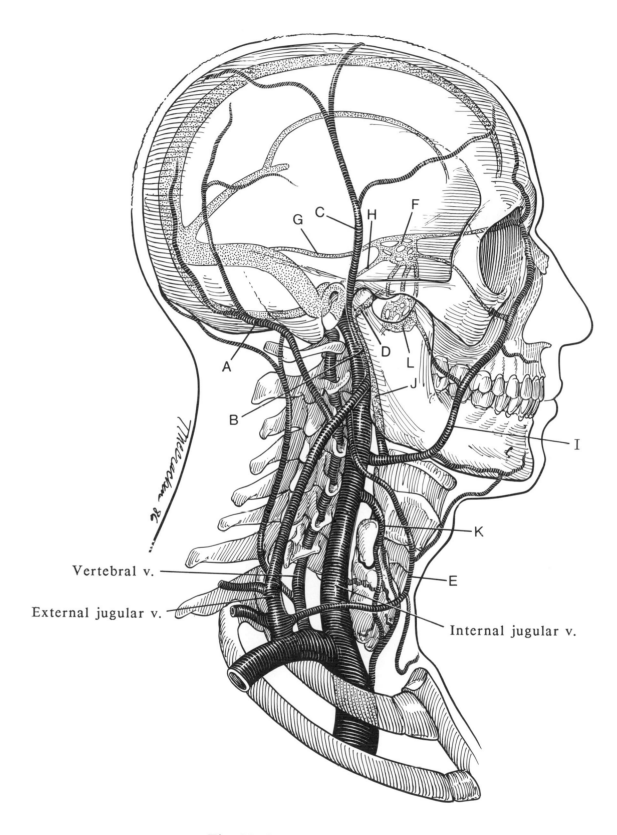

Vertebral v.

External jugular v.

Internal jugular v.

Fig. 11.10  Venous Drainage of Head

# UNIT FOUR: LOWER LIMB

## EXERCISE 12. BONES OF THE LOWER LIMB

As with the upper limb, the study of the lower limb begins with bones. You should become thoroughly familiar with these skeletal structures in order to further your understanding of lower limb function. Diagrams are provided to aid in identifying the following structures.

### I. Pelvis (Figures 12.1 and 12.2)

A. Each of the two coxal or "hip" bones consists developmentally of three separate bones: ilium, ischium, and pubis. Identify the approximate extent of each of these bones. The ilium is the most superior portion of the coxal bone and forms the superior portion of the the acetabulum (the deep cup-shaped cavity on the lateral aspect) and the "wings" rising and spreading from the main structure. The ischium forms the postero-inferior portion of the acetabulum and the lower posterior portion of the coxal bone. The pubis forms the anterior portion of the acetabulum and the anteromedial portion of the coxal bone. Find the following landmarks on the figures and label them appropriately.

### II. Ilium

A. **Iliac crest**

B. **Iliac fossa**

C. **Iliac tuberosity**

D. **Auricular surface**

E. **Anterior superior iliac spine**

F. **Anterior inferior iliac spine**

G. **Posterior superior iliac spine**

H. **Posterior inferior iliac spine**

I. **Inferior, anterior, and posterior gluteal lines**

### III. Ischium

J. **Body**

K. **Ramus**

L. **Ischial tuberosity**

M. **Ischial spine**

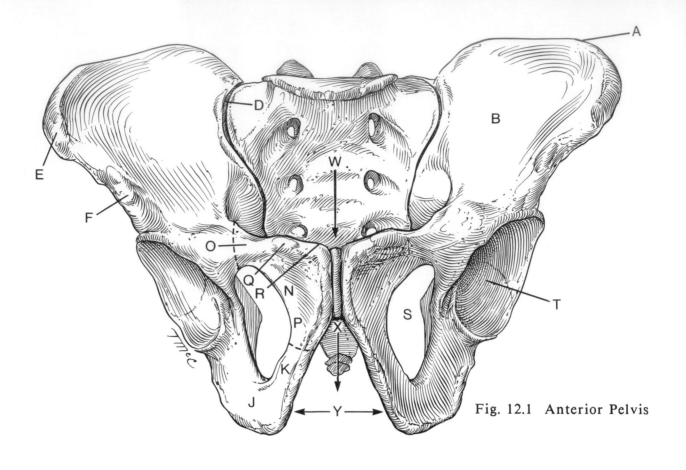

Fig. 12.1 Anterior Pelvis

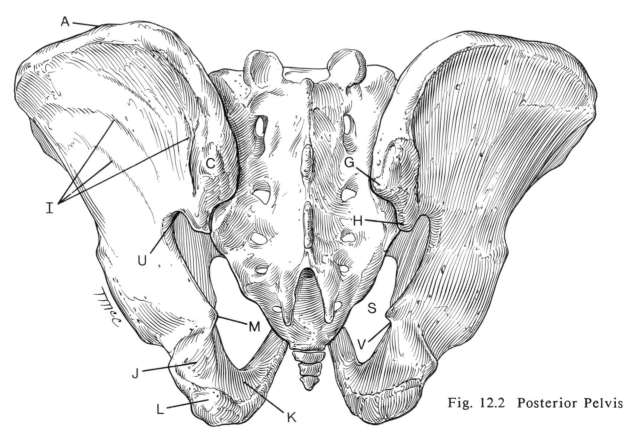

Fig. 12.2 Posterior Pelvis

IV. **Pubis**

    N.    **Body**

    O.    **Superior ramus**

    P.    **Inferior ramus**

    Q.    **Pubic tubercle**

    R.    **Pubic crest**

V. **Other Pelvic Features**

    S.    **Obturator foramen**

    T.    **Acetabulum**

    U.    **Greater sciatic notch**

    V.    **Lesser sciatic notch**

    W.    **Pelvic inlet**

    X.    **Pelvic outlet**

    Y.    **Pubic arch (angle)**

Before proceeding with the bones of the lower limb, you should review the landmarks of the sacrum (**Exercise 5**).

VI. **Femur (Figures 12.3 and 12.4)** - The femur is the longest bone in the body and may be conceptually divided into a shaft with neck and proximal and distal ends.

    A.    **Head**

    B.    **Neck**

    C.    **Greater trochanter**

    D.    **Lesser trochanter**

    E.    **Intertrochanteric crest (posterior)**

    F.    **Intertrochanteric line (anterior)**

    G.    **Gluteal tuberosity**

    H.    **Pectineal line**

    I.    **Linea aspera**

    J.    **Medial condyle and epicondyle**

K.     Lateral condyle and epicondyle

L.     Adductor tubercle

M.     Intercondylar fossa

N.     Patellar articular surface

## VII. Tibia (Figures 12.3 and 12.4)

O.     **Tibial tuberosity**

P.     **Medial condyle**

Q.     **Lateral condyle**

R.     **Intercondylar eminence**

S.     **Soleal line**

T.     **Medial malleollus**

U.     **Groove for tibialis posterior**

V.     **Fibular notch**

## VIII. Fibula (Figures 12.3 and 12.4)

W.     **Head**

X.     **Shaft**

Y.     **Lateral malleolus**

## IX. Foot (Figures 12.5 and 12.6)

### Tarsals

A.     **Calcaneus**

     1.    Sustentaculum tali

     2.    Tuber calcanei

     3.    Groove for flexor hallucis longus

B.     **Talus**

     4.    Head

     5.    Neck

     6.    Body

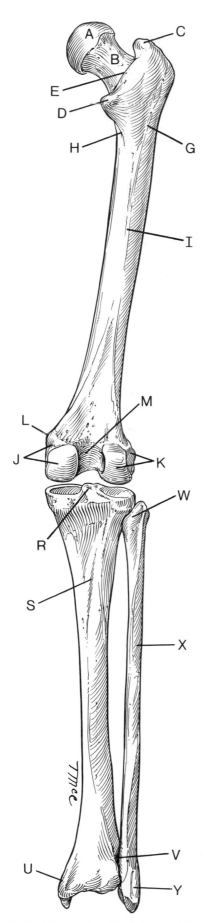

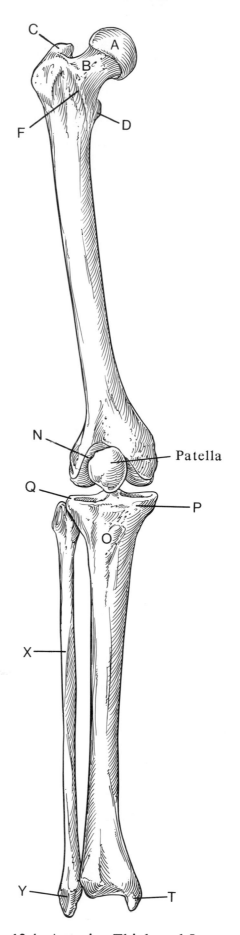

Fig. 12.3  Posterior Thigh and Leg          Fig. 12.4  Anterior Thigh and Leg

147

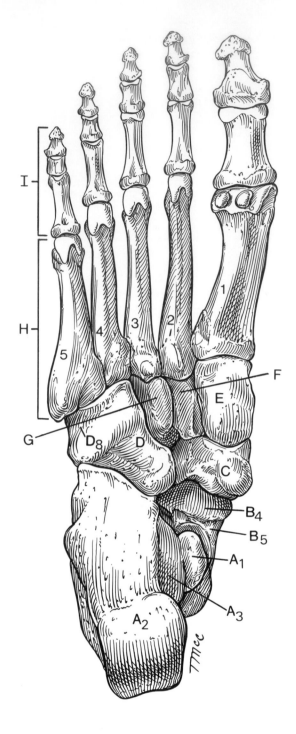

Fig. 12.5  Plantar Surface of Foot

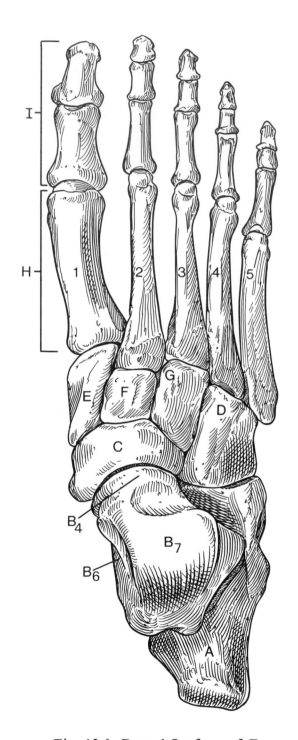

Fig. 12.6  Dorsal Surface of Foot

7.     Trochlea tali, with medial, lateral, and superior articular surfaces

C.    **Navicular**

D.    **Cuboid**

8.     Groove for peroneus longus

E.    **Medial cuneiform**

F.    **Intermediate cuneiform**

G.    **Lateral cuneiform**

**Metatarsals**

H.    **Metatarsals (5)** - numbered 1-5 from medial to lateral; each has a base (proximal), shaft, and head (distal)

**Phalanges**

I.    **Phalanges (14)** - also numbered 1-5 from medial to lateral; the great toe is similar to the thumb in having only two phalanges

## FOR REVIEW AND THOUGHT

Compare "equivalent" joints of the lower and upper limbs: hip and shoulder, knee and elbow, ankle and wrist. Which movements are similar and which are different? Why?

# NOTES

# EXERCISE 13.  GLUTEAL REGION;  LUMBOSACRAL PLEXUS

The gluteal region contains some powerful muscles used in locomotion, smaller muscles that function in rotation of the femur, and nerves traversing the buttocks to reach the lower limb.  Before beginning this exercise review the terminology from **Exercise 12** relating to the pelvis and femur.

## I.  Gluteal Muscles

Three pair of gluteal muscles take their proximal attachments off portions of the sacrum and ilium and attach distally to the femur.  They are arranged progressively anterior and deep to one another (Figures 13.1 and 13.2)

A.   **Gluteus maximus (                    )**

The gluteus maximus produces powerful extension at the hip, as in running or standing up from a seated position.  Like the trapezius and latissimus dorsi in the upper limb this muscle also serves to anchor the lower limb to the trunk. List the proximal and distal attachments below.

PA -

DA -

B.   **Gluteus medius (                    )**

This muscle is located deep and anterior to the gluteus maximus.  Its main action is to abduct the femur, but it also participates in medial rotation of the femur.  List the proximal and distal attachments.

PA -

DA -

C.   **Gluteus minimus (                    )**

The smallest of the three gluteal muscles is located deep and anterior to the gluteus medius.  It also functions primarily in abduction of the femur with a secondary action in medial rotation.

PA -

DA -

Now that you have studied these muscles and their attachments, use the space below to describe their roles in locomotion.

151

## II. Deep Rotators

When the gluteal muscles are cut and reflected (Figures 13.1 and 13.2), a group of small muscles may be seen. Because all of these muscles function in lateral rotation of the femur they are referred to as the deep, or short, rotator group.

D.   **Piriformis (                    )**

This muscle has its proximal attachment off the anterior surface of the sacrum and passes out the greater sciatic foramen (dividing the foramen into superior and inferior portions) to have its distal attachment where?

DA -

The piriformis is also important as a landmark because the sciatic nerve usually exits the pelvis immediately inferior to this muscle. The sciatic nerve is a branch of the lumbosacral plexus and will be described below.

E.   **Obturator internus (                    )**

As implied by its name this muscle takes proximal attachment of the inner surface of the obturator membrane and the ischiopubic rami surrounding the obturator foramen. What is its distal attachment?

DA -

Notice the course taken by this muscle. Between what two landmarks does it exit the pelvis? _____ and

_____.

F.   **Superior gemellus (                    )**

The belly of this muscle is seen immediately superior to the obturator internus. Its distal attachment is into the tendon of the obturator internus. What is the proximal attachment of the superior gemellus?

PA -

G.   **Inferior gemellus (                    )**

As you might guess, the inferior gemellus is found immediately inferior to the obturator internus and has a similar distal attachment as its superior counterpart. List the proximal attachment of this muscle.
PA -

H.   **Quadratus femoris (                    )**

Quadrate in shape, this muscle is found inferior to the inferior gemellus. Its distal attachment is on the quadrate line on the posterior aspect of the greater trochanter. What is its proximal attachment?

PA -

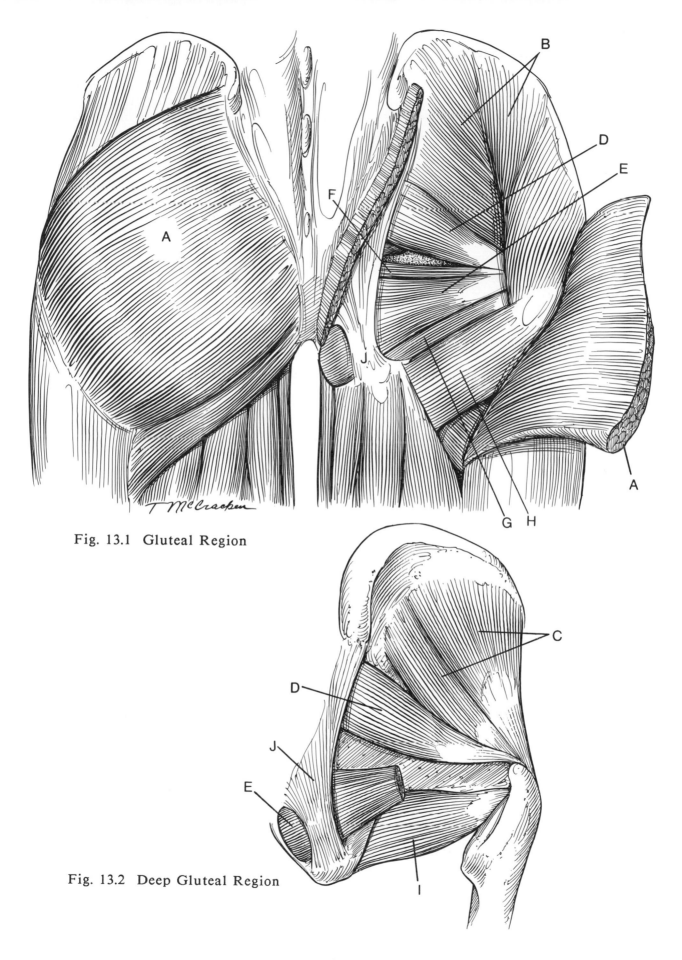

Fig. 13.1  Gluteal Region

Fig. 13.2  Deep Gluteal Region

153

I.    Obturator externus (                              )

This muscle is located deep to the quadratus femoris.  It too is a lateral rotator of the thigh with a distal attachment on the trochanteric fossa.  Given the description of the proximal attachment of the obturator internus (see E, previous page), list the proximal attachment of the externus.

PA -

J.    **Sacrotuberous ligament**

This ligament attaches superiorly to the the dorsal surface of the sacrum and the coccyx.  Its inferior attachment is to the ischial tuberosity.

K.    **Sacropsinous ligament**

Lying deep to the sacrotuberous ligament, its attachments are the sacrum and coccyx medially and the ischial spine laterally.  The sacrotuberous and sacrospinous ligaments convert the greater and lesser sciatic notches into foramina, with the sacrospinous ligament demarcating these two foramina.

III.    **Lumbosacral Plexus (Figure 13.3)**

The lumbosacral plexus is formed by ventral primary rami of lumbar and sacral spinal nerves.  The branches of $L_1$ - $L_3$ and part of $L_4$ form the lumbar portion of the plexus, which lies, with its roots, within the psoas major muscle.  Like the brachial plexus, anterior and posterior divisions are given off, which then join to form nerves.  Because of the medial rotation of the lower limb during embryonic development, nerves formed by posterior divisions come to supply anteriorly placed muscles and nerves formed by anterior divisions come to supply posteriorly placed muscles.  The basic concept of posterior nerves supplying extensors and anterior nerves supplying flexors still holds, however.

A.    **Lumbar Plexus**

**Nerves from anterior divisions**

1.    Ilioinguinal nerve ($L_1$) - sensory to the external genitalia; motor to abdominal wall.

2.    Genitofemoral nerve ($L_1$, $L_2$) - divides into genital and femoral branches; the genital branch travels with the spermatic cord into the scrotum (or with the ligamentum teres into the labia majora in the female); supplies the cremaster muscle and is sensory to the skin of the external genitalia and medial thigh.

      The femoral branch is sensory to the thigh in the area of the femoral triangle.

3.    Obturator nerve ($L_2$, $L_3$, $L_4$) - motor to the muscles of the adductor (medial) compartment of the thigh.

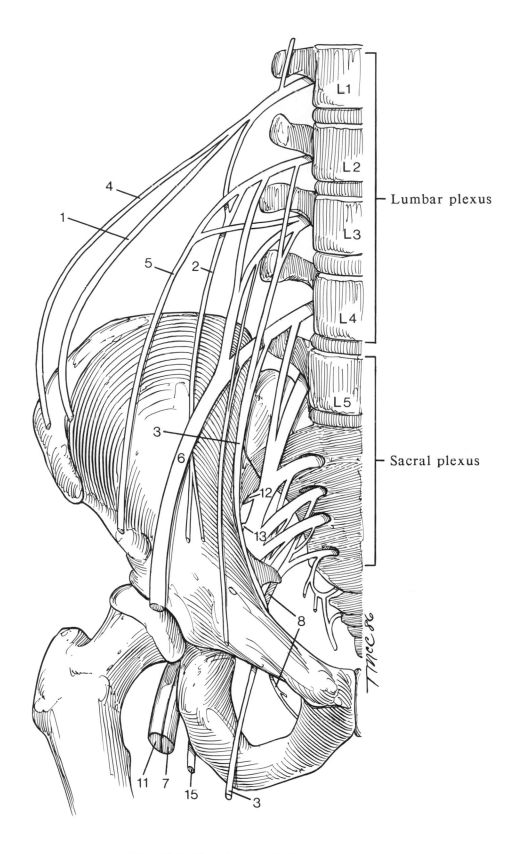

Fig. 13.3  Lumbosacral Plexus

155

### Nerves from posterior divisions

4. Iliohypogastric nerve ($L_1$) - supplies the skin of the gluteal region via a lateral branch and the skin over the inguinal ligament via an anterior branch.

5. Lateral femoral cutaneous nerve ($L_2$, $L_3$) - sensory to the lateral thigh.

6. Femoral nerve ($L_2$, $L_3$, $L_4$) - motor to the iliacus, psoas major, psoas minor and the muscles of the anterior thigh.

The remainder of $L_4$ ventral ramus and all of $L_5$ join to form the lumbosacral trunk, connecting the lumbar and sacral plexuses.

B. **Sacral Plexus**

### Nerves from anterior divisions

7. Tibial ($L_5$, $S_1$, $S_2$, $S_3$) - motor to most of the posterior thigh; posterior leg; and plantar surface of the foot.

8. Pudendal ($S_2$, $S_3$, $S_4$) - sensory to genitalia; motor to perineal muscles and sphincter urethrae, external anal sphincter and levator ani.

9. Nerve to the superior gemellus and obturator internus ($L_5$, $S_1$, $S_2$).

10. Nerve to the quadratus femoris and inferior gemellus ($L_4$, $L_5$, $S_1$).

### Nerves from posterior divisions

11. Common peroneal nerve ($L_4$, $L_5$, $S_1$, $S_2$) - motor to one-half of one muscle in the posterior thigh, muscles of lateral leg, anterior leg, and dorsum of the foot.

12. Superior gluteal nerve ($L_4$, $L_5$, $S_1$) - motor to the gluteus medius, gluteus minimus, and tensor fascia latae.

13. Inferior gluteal nerve ($L_5$, $S_1$, $S_2$) - motor to the gluteus maximus.

14. Nerve to the piriformis ($S_1$, $S_2$).

The posterior femoral cutaneous nerve is formed by posterior divisions of $S_1$, and $S_2$ and anterior divisions of $S_2$ and $S_3$.

15. Posterior femoral cutaneous ($S_1$, $S_2$, $S_3$) - sensory to the posterior thigh.

The tibial and common peroneal nerves are usually physically united within a connective tissue sheath to form the sciatic nerve.

Use Figures 13.4 and 13.5 to trace the major nerves of the plexus to their destination in the lower limb.

## FOR REVIEW AND THOUGHT

Review the passage of the "sciatic" nerve through the gluteal region. Might this nerve be endangered in gluteal injections? Where should such injections be administered?

With your laboratory or study partners begin to discuss the consequences of nerve injury in the pelvic or gluteal regions. What functional losses might be seen in the limb?

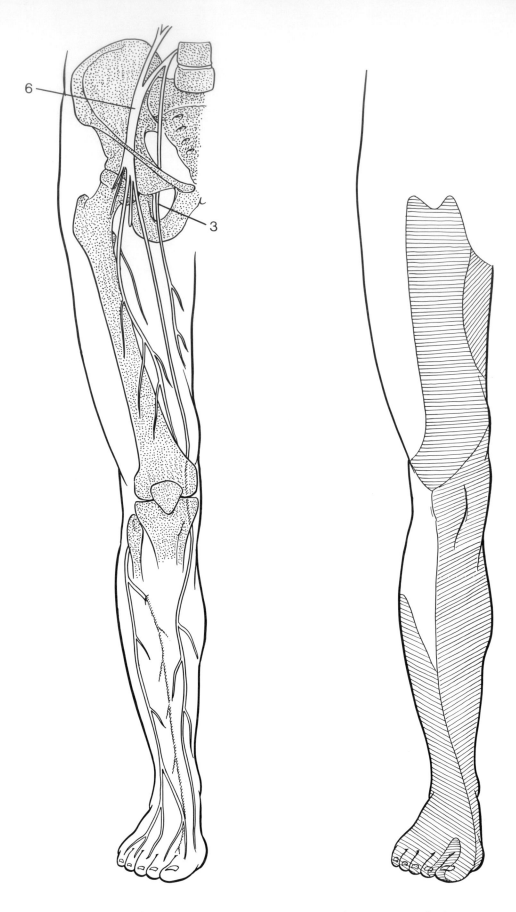

Fig. 13.4  Nerve Supply, Anterior Lower Limb

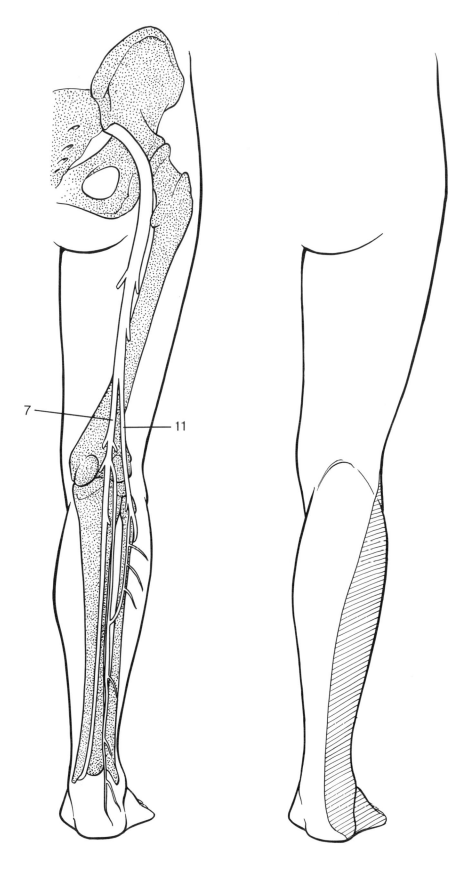

Fig. 13.5  Nerve Supply, Posterior Lower Limb

159

# NOTES

# EXERCISE 14. THIGH AND KNEE

The thigh is conveniently arranged in compartments by deep extensions of the fascia lata (deep fascia of the thigh). These extensions attach to the linea aspera of the femur and divide the thigh into anterior (extensor), posterior (flexor), and medial (adductor) compartments. Each of these compartments is innervated via one of the motor nerves of the lumbosacral plexus.

## I. Anterior Thigh (Figure 14.1)

### A. Quadriceps femoris (          )

This four headed muscle is the main occupant of the anterior thigh. One of these four heads has a proximal attachment on the ilium. Which one? _____ The other three heads have their proximal attachments on the shaft of the femur. List the specific proximal attachment of each head below.

1. Rectus femoris

   PA -

2. Vastus lateralis

   PA -

3. Vastus medialis

   PA -

4. Vastus intermedius

   PA -

What is the distal attachment of the quadriceps femoris as a whole?

_____

Given this, what is the function of the quadriceps femoris?

_____

### B. Sartorius (          )

This is the most superficial muscle of the anterior thigh, taking an oblique course from superolateral to inferomedial. List the proximal and distal attachments below.

PA -

DA -

This long flat muscle takes its name from the Latin word for tailor, because of the tailor's habit of sitting cross-legged while working. Contraction of the sartorius produces the movements necessary to sit cross-legged. Do this yourself and describe the actions of the sartorius.

The sartorius also forms the lateral boundary of an area known as the femoral triangle. The medial border of this triangle is formed by the adductor longus. Study Figure 14.2 to deduce the superior boundary of this triangle.

---

Two muscles form the floor of the femoral triangle, the iliopsoas and pectineus.

C.   **Iliopsoas (                    )**

This is the more lateral of the two muscles. It is, in reality, a compound muscle formed by the union of the psoas major and iliacus. This union provides for a common distal attachment. List the proximal attachments and distal attachment below.

PA (Iliacus) -

PA (Psoas major) -

DA (Iliopsoas) -

From such attachments, what is the function of the iliopsoas?

---

D.   **Pectineus (                    )**

Discrepancy exists whether this muscle should be listed with the anterior or medial thigh muscles. The pectineus functions as both an adductor and a flexor of the thigh, thus the confusion. Because of this it is usually innervated by both of the nerves supplying the anterior and medial compartments. List the attachments of this muscle below.

PA -

DA -

The femoral triangle contains several important structures (Figure 14.2). From lateral to medial these are the femoral nerve, femoral artery, femoral vein, and femoral canal (empty space containing lymph nodes and lymphatic vessels). Notice the underlined letters form the word NAVEL. Use this acronym to help you remember the contents of the femoral triangle.

Within the triangle the femoral nerve branches, the femoral artery gives off the deep femoral artery, and the femoral vein receives drainage from the great saphenous vein.

E.   **Tensor fascia latae (                         )**

The tensor fascia latae is the most anterior of the muscles on the lateral surface of the ilium. Its proximal attachment is off the most anterior portion of the iliac crest and the notch between the anterior and superior iliac spines.

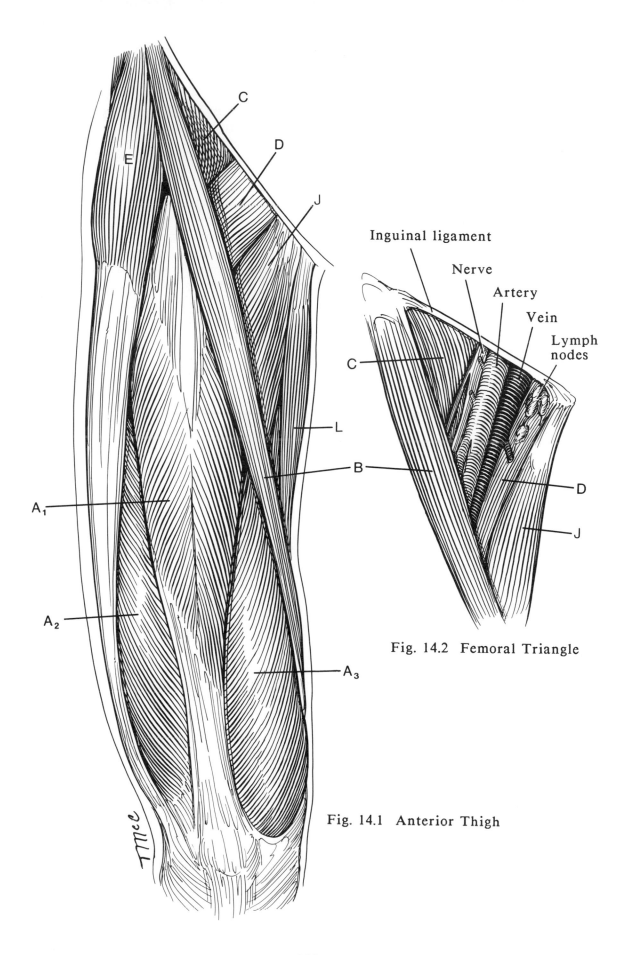

C

D

E

J

A₁

A₂

A₃

B

L

Inguinal ligament

Nerve

Artery

Vein

Lymph
nodes

C

D

J

Fig. 14.2  Femoral Triangle

Fig. 14.1  Anterior Thigh

Distally this muscle attaches into the iliotibial tract, which also serves as the distal attachment of part of the gluteus maximus.

The iliotibial tract is laterally placed on the thigh and runs from the ilium to the lateral condyle of the tibia. This tract is a thickened portion of the fascia lata, a bandaging layer of fascia enveloping the thigh.

## II. Posterior Thigh (Figure 14.3)

The muscles of the posterior thigh are often called the "hamstrings."

F. **Biceps Femoris (**             **)**

This is the most lateral of the posterior muscles and is composed of long and short heads. The long head shows a common proximal attachment with the other posterior muscles from the ischial tuberosity. What is the proximal attachment of the short head? _____
What is the distal attachment of the biceps femoris?

DA -

G. **Semitendinosus (**             **)**

The distal portion of this muscle is a long slender tendon. Into what does this tendon have its distal attachment?

DA -

H. **Semimembranosus (**             **)**

The proximal portion of this muscle is a flattened membranous tendon. What is the distal attachment of this muscle?

DA -

Nerve supply to those portions of the "hamstring" group with proximal attachment on the ischial tuberosity is provided by the tibial portion of the sciatic nerve while the common peroneal portion of the sciatic supplies those muscles with proximal attachment elsewhere. Given this, fill in the nerve supply in the brackets next to each muscle.

I. **Adductor magnus (**             **)**

Like the pectineus, the adductor magnus may be described with two groups: posterior and medial. Because of its proximal attachment from the ischial ramus and ischial tuberosity, it functions as both an adductor and a "hamstring." Write in the nerve supply to this muscle and list its distal attachment.

DA -

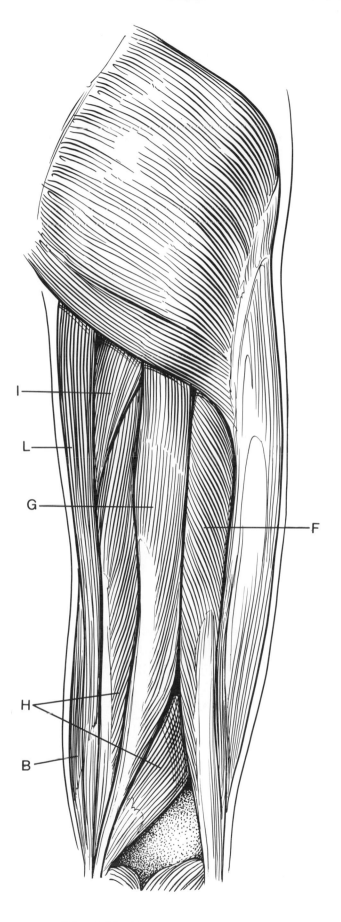

Fig. 14.3  Posterior Thigh

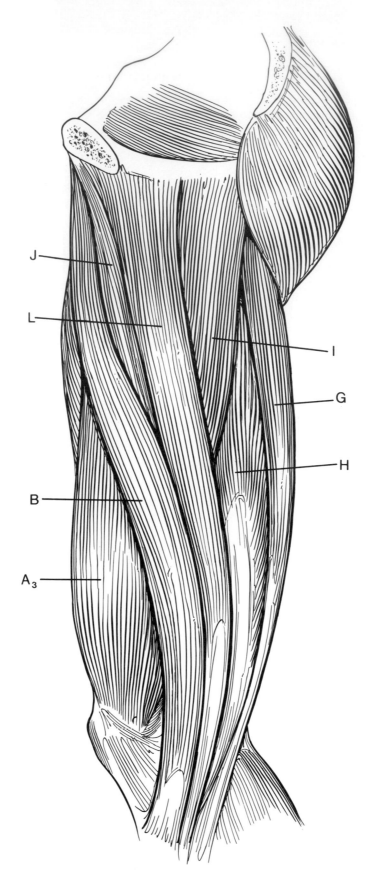

Fig. 14.4  Medial Thigh

166

## III. Medial Thigh (Figure 14.4)

Three adductor muscles are named:  magnus, longus, and brevis.  The adductor magnus has already been studied.

J.   **Adductor longus (                    )**

This is the most anterior of the three adductors and has been previously described as the medial boundary of the femoral triangle.  It takes proximal attachment from the body of the pubis just inferior to the pubic tubercle. What is its distal attachment?

DA -

K.   **Adductor brevis (                    )**

Found deep to the adductor longus it has a similar proximal attachment, and a distal attachment on the superior end of the linea aspera and on a line between the linea aspera and lesser trochanter.

What is the nerve supply of the medial (adductor) compartment?
_____ This
nerve splits into anterior and posterior branches as it leaves the pelvis.  These branches are sandwiched between the adductor muscles as follows:

Adductor longus

Anterior branch

Adductor brevis

Posterior branch

Adductor magnus

L.   **Gracilis (                    )**

This long slender muscle takes proximal attachment from the body of the pubis. What is the distal attachment of the gracilis?

DA -

Three muscles have distal attachment on the anterior surface of the medial condyle of the tibia.  This attachment is known as the "pes anserine" (foot of the goose).  What three muscles are these?

_____

_____

_____

What is significant about these three muscles?

167

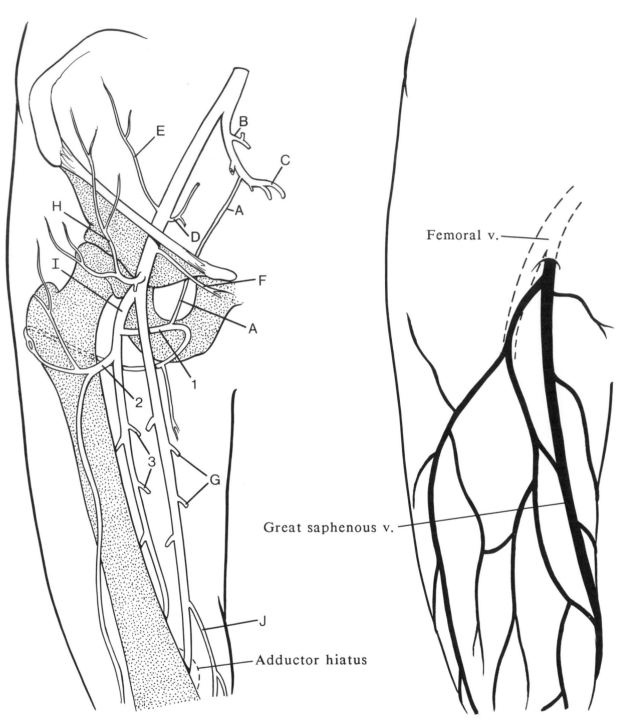

Fig. 14.5  Arterial Supply,
Anterior Thigh

Fig. 14.6  Venous Drainage,
Anterior Thigh

Femoral v.

Great saphenous v.

Adductor hiatus

## IV. Course of the Femoral Artery and Vein

As these vessels leave the apex of the femoral triangle they lie deep to the sartorius muscle and upon the anterior surface of the adductor magnus. This is known as the subsartorial or adductor canal (also called Hunter's canal). In their course through the canal, the vessels are accompanied by the saphenous nerve, a sensory branch of the femoral nerve. The canal ends at the adductor hiatus (a gap in the adductor magnus), through which the vessels pass to reach the popliteal fossa and become the popliteal vessels while the saphenous nerve passes superficially (Figures 14.5 and 14.6). (An outline of arterial and venous structures is presented on pp. 191-192.)

## V. Knee Joint (Figures 14.7 and 14.8)

Skeletally the knee is quite unstable: two large, rounded femoral condyles sliding and rolling upon two shallow tibial condyles. Structurally, however, the knee is sound because of surrounding muscles, a strong articular capsule, and integrity of internal and external ligaments.

When the quadriceps tendon and patella are removed and the joint is flexed, the anterior portion of the knee joint is exposed (Figure 14.7). Several structures may be seen clearly.

A.   **Medial meniscus**

B.   **Lateral meniscus**

The menisci are fibrocartilagenous pads that function to absorb shock and to slightly deepen the tibial articular surfaces for the femoral condyles. The menisci are held to the tibia by coronary ligaments.

C.   **Coronary ligament**

D.   **Transverse genicular ligament** - connecting the two menisci

E.   **Anterior cruciate ligament** - passing from the medial surface of the lateral femoral condyle to the anterior portion of the intercondylar eminence of the tibia

F.   **Fibular collateral ligament**

G.   **Tibial collateral ligament**

The tibial collateral ligament has a physical attachment to the medial meniscus. The fibular collateral ligament has no such attachment to the lateral meniscus.

Figure 14.8 shows the joint in an extended position and allows visualization of posterior structures.

H.   **Popliteus muscle (                    )**

The proximal attachment of this muscle is the lateral condyle of the femur. What is its distal attachment?

The tendon of the popliteus intervenes between the fibular collateral ligament and the lateral meniscus, preventing their union.

I. **Posterior cruciate ligament** - passing from the lateral surface of the medial femoral condyle to the posterior portion of the intercondylar eminence of the tibia.

J. **Posterior meniscofemoral ligament** - passes from the posterior portion of the lateral meniscus to the lateral surface of the medial femoral condyle immediately posterior to the posterior cruciate.

The four major ligaments of the knee limit excessive movement (i.e., provide stability). The collateral ligaments limit lateral movement of the joint. The cruciate ligaments limit movement of the tibia in the direction of their name.

The tibial collateral ligament and lateral meniscus are usually injured together because of their physical attachment. Often, in situations such as clipping in football, the anterior cruciate ligament is also damaged. This threesome is then referred to as the "terrible triad."

**FOR REVIEW AND THOUGHT**

Discuss the action of the popliteus muscle in a free limb vs. a limb bearing weight.

Think about and discuss further the significance of the pes anserine.

Review the structure of the knee, focusing your attention on the bones and ligaments involved in the joint. Discuss the factors leading to stability or instability of the joint.

The lower limb is adapted for support and the upper limb for mobility, yet they are similar in overall design. List below the similarities and differences you have found so far between the limbs.

Similarities:

Differences:

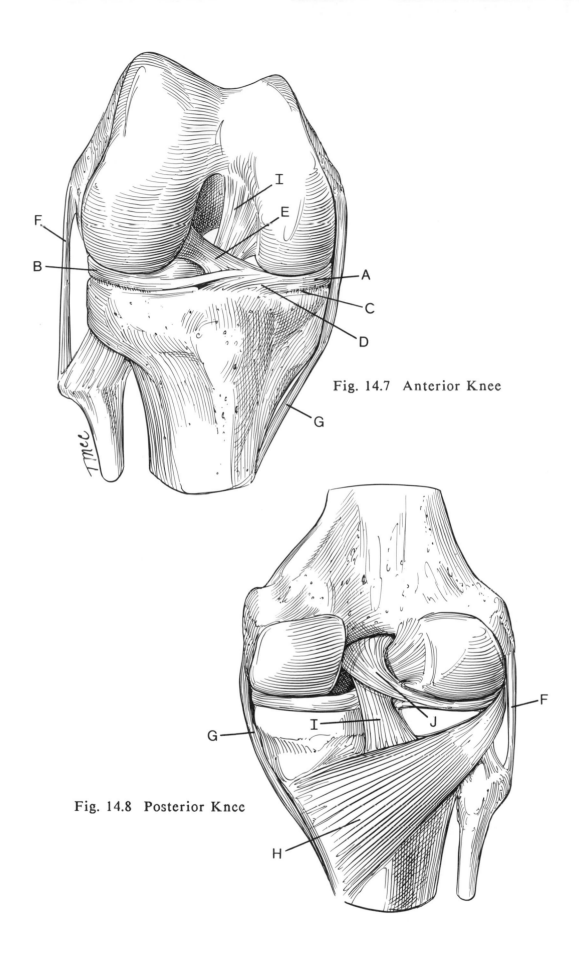

Fig. 14.7  Anterior Knee

Fig. 14.8  Posterior Knee

# NOTES

# EXERCISE 15.  LEG AND FOOT

The leg is divided into three compartments, each with its own nerve.  An interosseus membrane between the tibia and fibula separates the anterior (extensor) and posterior (flexor) compartments.  The lateral (peroneal) compartment is bounded by anterior and posterior fascial septa passing deeply from the crural fascia and attaching to the fibula.

Two specific terms are used to describe movements at the ankle (talo-crural) joint: dorsiflexion and plantar flexion.  Dorsiflexion is the movement of the dorsal surface of the foot and the anterior surface of the leg toward one another.  Plantar flexion is the opposite movement.  Inversion (turning in) and eversion (turning out) of the foot occurs at the joints between the calcaneus and cuboid and the talus and navicular.  The two joints are nearly in line horizontally and form what is known as the "transverse tarsal joint" (Figures 12.5 and 12.6).

I.  Leg

   Anterior compartment (Figure 15.1)

   A.  **Tibialis anterior (                    )**

   The proximal attachment of this muscle is from the lateral condyle and lateral surface of the shaft of the tibia.  What is the distal attachment?

   DA -


   B.  **Extensor hallucis longus (                    )**

   The fibula and interosseus membrane serve as the proximal attachment of the extensor hallucis longus.  List its distal attachment below.

   DA -


   What was the equivalent term for hallucis in the upper limb?

   _____

   C.  **Extensor digitorum longus (                    )**

   This muscle takes proximal attachment from the lateral condyle of the tibia, shaft of the fibula, and interosseus membranes.  What is its distal attachment?

   DA -


   What muscle in the upper limb has a similar distal attachment?

   _____

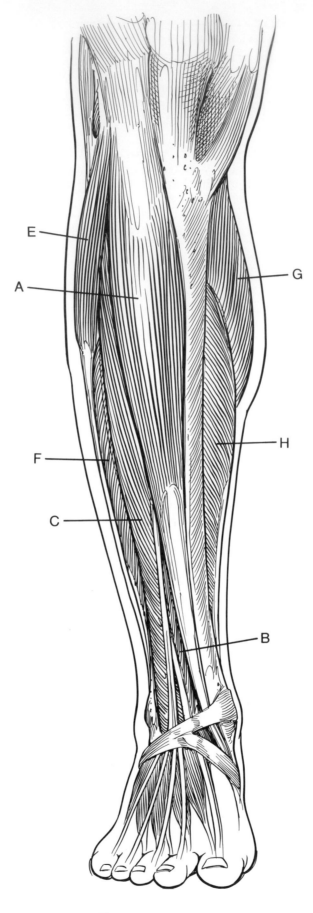

Fig. 15.1  Anterior Leg

174

D. **Peroneus tertius (**                 **) (Figure 15.2)**

The peroneus tertius has a proximal attachment on the distal fibula and interosseus membrane. Its distal attachment is to the base of the fifth metatarsal. How does this distal attachment differ from that of the extensor digitorum longus? _____

_____

Each of the muscles of the anterior compartment has a specific action because of the various distal attachments. List the specific action of each below.

Tibialis anterior -

Extensor hallucis longus -

Extensor digitorum longus -

Peroneus tertius -

In addition, these muscles have one action in common. That action is

_____

**Lateral Compartment (Figure 15.2)**

Peroneus is derived from the Latin word for fibula and describes the proximal attachment of both muscles in this compartment. The distal attachments vary considerably, however!

E. **Peroneus longus (**            **)**

DA -

F. **Peroneus brevis (**            **)**

DA -

These muscles have two actions in common. One of these actions occurs at the ankle and one at the transverse tarsal joint. What are these actions?

_____

Explain why these muscles have such an action at the ankle? _____

_____

Why doesn't the peroneus tertius have the same actions? _____

_____

175

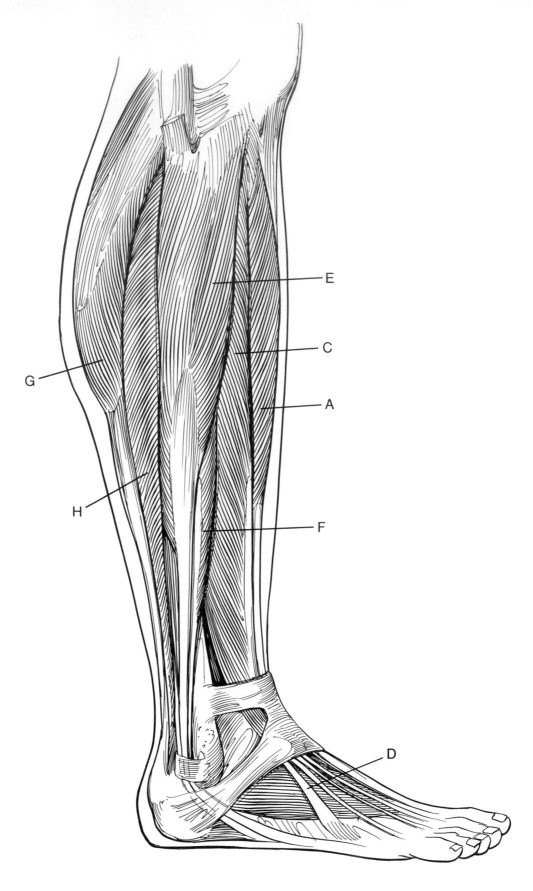

Fig. 15.2  Lateral Leg

176

## Posterior Compartment (Figures 15.3 and 15.4)

### Superficial Group (Figure 15.3)

The superficial group is composed of gastrocnemius, soleus, and plantaris. The gastrocnemius takes its proximal attachment off the femur via two heads and the soleus off the posterior surface of the fibula and tibia. These two muscles have a common distal attachment and are sometimes grouped as the "triceps surae." List the specific attachments below.

G.　**Gastrocnemius (** 　　　　　　　**)**

Lateral Head

PA -

DA -

Medial Head

PA -

DA -

H.　**Soleus (** 　　　　　　**)**

PA -

DA -

I.　**Plantaris (** 　　　　　**)**

The belly of this small muscle is seen superior to the lateral head of the gastrocnemius. Its tendon is conspicuously long and slender and is found along the medial border of the common tendon of the gastrocnemius and soleus.

PA -

DA -

Deep Group (Figure 15.4)

As with the forearm muscles, the deeper lying leg muscles have their action on more distal portions of the limb.

J.   **Flexor hallucis longus (                    )**

This muscle has its proximal attachment off the inferior posterior fibula and interosseus membrane.  The belly of the muscle converges to a tendon that leaves a deep groove on the inferior surface of the sustentaculum tali.  What is the distal attachment of this muscle?

DA -


K.   **Flexor digitorum longus (                    )**

From its proximal attachment on the inferior posterior tibia this muscle narrows to a tendon that crosses the flexor hallucis longus tendon on the plantar surface of the sustentaculum tali before splitting into four tendinous slips to the lateral four toes.  List the specific distal attachment below.

DA -


L.   **Tibialis posterior (                    )**

Besides what is implied by its name, this muscle also has proximal  attachment to the fibula and interosseus membrane.  The tendon of the muscle leaves a prominent groove on the posterior surface of the medial malleolus.  The distal attachment is extensive:   into the tuberosity of the navicular, three cuneiforms, cuboid, and the bases of metatarsals 2, 3, and 4.

Each of the muscles of the posterior compartment has a specific action based upon attachments.  List these specific actions.

Gastrocnemius -


Soleus -


Plantaris -


Flexor hallucis longus -


Flexor digitorum longus -


Tibialis posterior -


What one action do all these muscles have in common? _____

_____

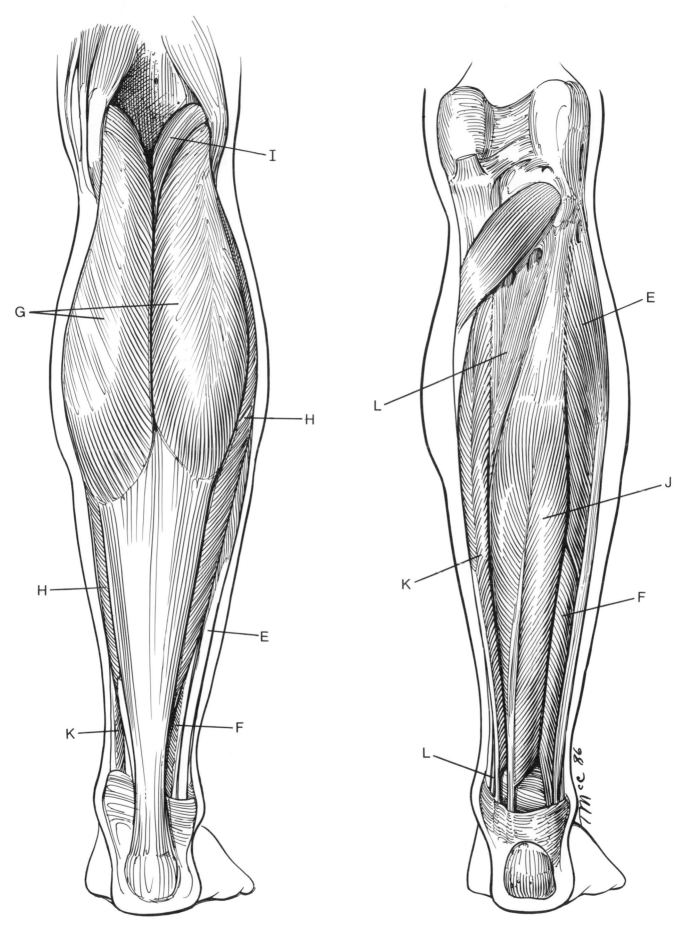

Fig. 15.3  Posterior Leg,
Superficial Group

179

Fig. 15.4  Posterior Leg,
Deep Group

## II. Foot

### Dorsum (Figure 15.5)

Most of the dorsum of the foot is occupied by the tendons of the extrinsic muscles of the anterior compartment of the leg. These tendons are held in place by the extensor retinaculum. Only one intrinsic muscle is present, the extensor digitorum brevis.

M.   **Extensor retinaculum**

N.   **Extensor digitorum brevis (**           **)**

Note the distal attachment of this muscle. How does it differ from that of extensor digitorum longus? _____

_____

### Plantar Surface

The muscles of the plantar surface of the foot are arranged and described in layers. The need to learn specific attachments of these muscles will be determined by educational objectives of a particular course. The concentration here will be on function, innervation, and comparison with the hand.

### First layer (Figure 15.6)

O.   **Abductor hallucis (**           **)**

P.   **Flexor digitorum brevis (**           **)**

Q.   **Abductor digiti minimi (**           **)**

The function of these muscles is obvious from their name. Into what phalanx of the toes would you expect the tendons of the flexor digitorum brevis to attach?

_____

### Second and third layers (Figure 15.7)

R.   **Quadratus plantae (**           **)**

Through its distal attachment into the tendon of the flexor digitorum longus, this muscle aids in flexing the toes and in correcting medial deviation of such flexion because of the angle at which the flexor digitorum longus tendon passes through the foot.

S.   **Tendon of flexor digitorum longus**

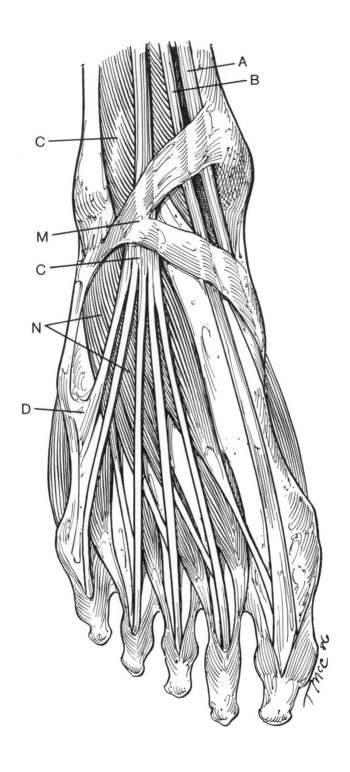

Fig. 15.5  Dorsal Foot

181

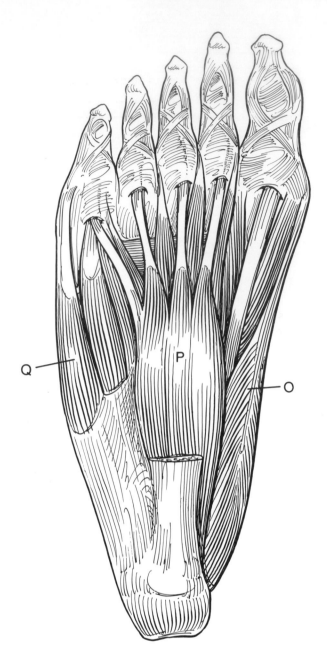

Fig. 15.6  Superficial Plantar Foot

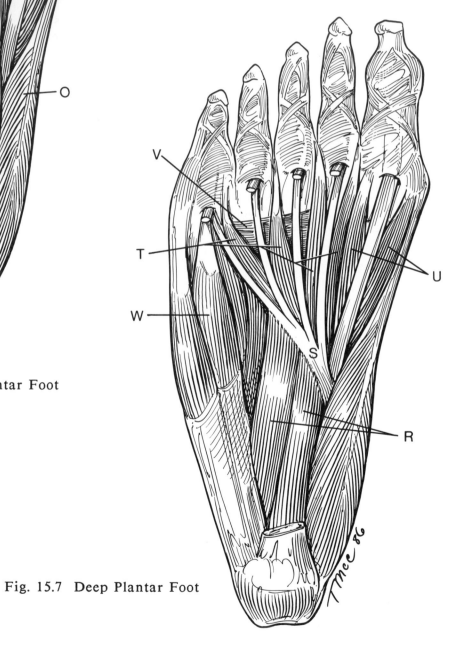

Fig. 15.7  Deep Plantar Foot

T.   **Lumbricals (                              )**

Four lumbricals arise from the medial sides of the tendons of flexor digitorum longus.  How is this different from the case in the hand?  _____

_____

Why might this be so?  _____

U.   **Flexor hallucis brevis (                    )**

V.   **Adductor hallucis (                    )**

W.   **Flexor digiti minimi brevis (                        )**

**Fourth layer (Figures 15.8 and 15.9)**

The fourth layer of the foot is composed of the interossei muscles.  Three plantar and four dorsal interossei are present, as was true in the hand.  The line about which ab- and adduction is defined is the middle of the second digit.  What was it in the hand?  _____

X.   **Plantar interossei**

Y.   **Dorsal interossei**

III.   **Neural Supply to the Leg and Foot**

As mentioned at the outset of this exercise, the compartments of the leg are each provided with a motor nerve.  The common peroneal portion of the sciatic nerve moves laterally in the popliteal fossa and curves around the neck of the fibula. Within the peroneus longus it splits into superficial and deep peroneal nerves, which are distributed as shown in Figures 13.4 and 15.10.

A.   **Superficial peroneal** - motor to the lateral compartment and sensory to the lower anterior leg and nearly all of the dorsum of the foot.

B.   **Deep peroneal** - motor to the anterior compartment and sensory to a small area between the first and second toes.

The tibial portion of the sciatic nerve continues on a straight course through the posterior compartment, lying between the superficial and deep groups and supplying all the muscles of the posterior compartment.  At the medial malleolus it splits into medial and lateral plantar nerves which supply the plantar surface of the foot (Figures 13.5 and 15.11).

C.   **Medial plantar** - motor to abductor hallucis, flexor digitorum brevis, and the first lumbrical; sensory to the medial three and one-half digits (Figure 15.11).

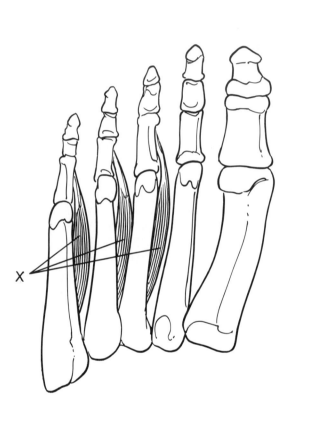

Fig. 15.8  Plantar View

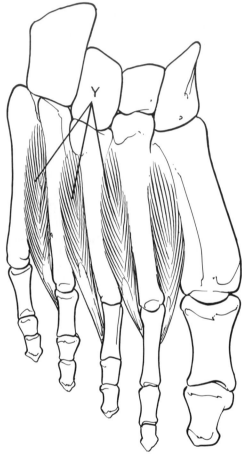

Fig. 15.9  Dorsal View

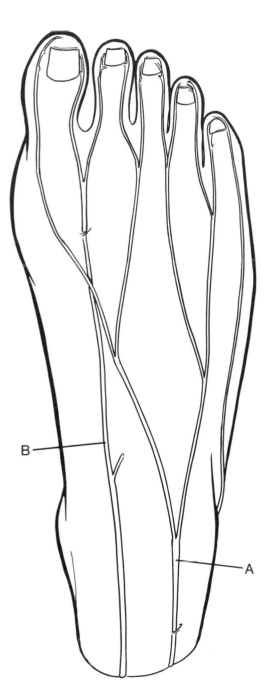

Fig. 15.10 Nerve Supply,
Dorsum of Foot

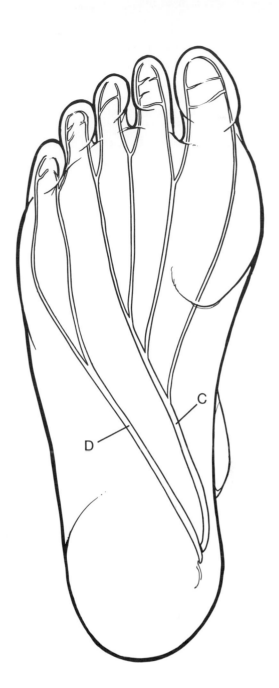

Fig. 15.11 Nerve Supply, Plantar
Surface of Foot

D.   **Lateral plantar** - motor to all other plantar muscles and sensory to the lateral one and one-half digits (Figure 15.11).

Now return to each of the muscles studied in this exercise and write the nerve supply in the brackets provided.

## IV. Vascular Structures in the Leg and Foot

### Arterial Supply

The arterial supply is similar except that the lateral compartment does not contain an artery.   Inferior to the knee the popliteal artery splits into anterior and posterior tibial arteries, and the posterior tibial subsequently gives off the peroneal artery (Figures 15.12 - 15.14).

> **Anterior tibial artery** - descends along the anterior surface of the interosseus membrane in company with the deep peroneal nerve; it is continued onto the dorsum of the foot as the dorsalis pedis.

P.   **Dorsalis pedis**

> **Posterior tibial artery** - descends in the posterior compartment between the superficial and deep groups; its major branch, the peroneal, remains in the posterior compartment, supplying the lateral portion of the compartment as well as sending branches to the lateral compartment.

Q.   **Peroneal**

> The terminal branches of the posterior tibial artery are the medial and lateral plantar arteries.  They accompany the nerves of the same name.

R.   **Medial plantar**

S.   **Lateral plantar**

> The lateral plantar artery joins with the deep branch of the dorsalis pedis to form the plantar arch.

### Venous Drainage

The lower limbs are supplied with both superficial and deep veins.   The deep veins accompany the named arteries, usually in pairs:  venae comitantes.  Two important superficial veins are present (Figures 15.12, 15.13).

> **Great saphenous** - begins on the medial side of the dorsal venous arch of the foot and ascends anterior to the medial malleolus, along the medial leg, behind the medial condyles of the tibia and femur, and along the medial thigh.  It terminates by emptying into the femoral vein in the femoral triangle.

> **Lesser saphenous** - begins on the lateral side of the dorsal venous arch of the foot and ascends posterior to the lateral malleolus, along the middle posterior leg to the popliteal fossa, where it terminates by emptying into the popliteal vein.

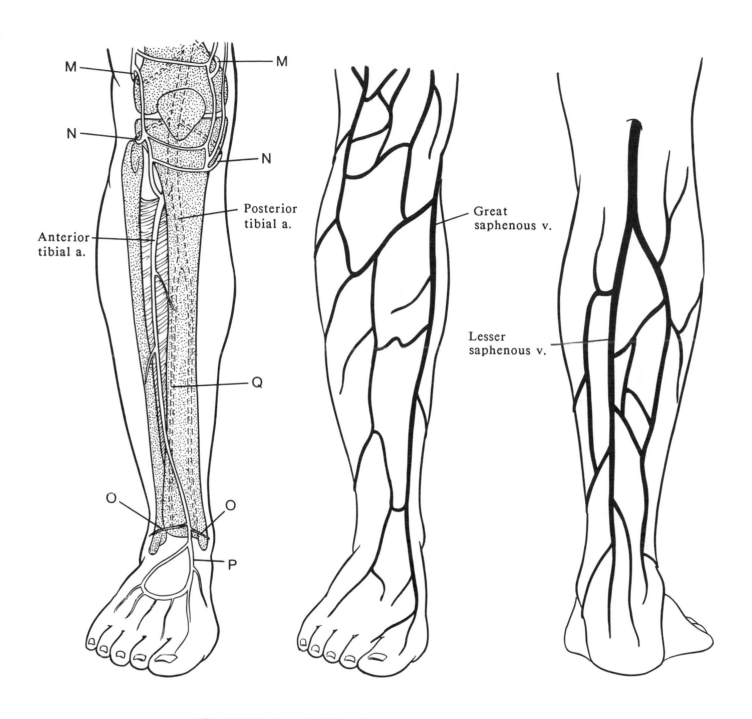

Fig. 15.12  Arterial Supply and Venous Drainage Leg

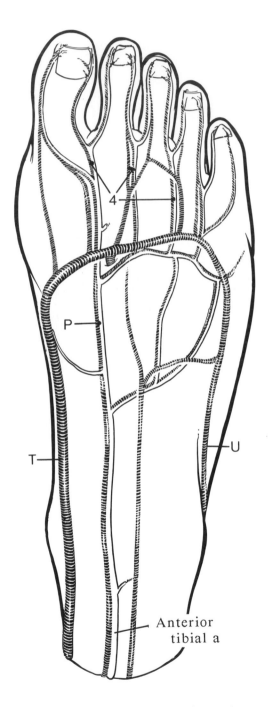

Fig. 15.13  Arterial Supply and
Venous Drainage,
Dorsum of Foot

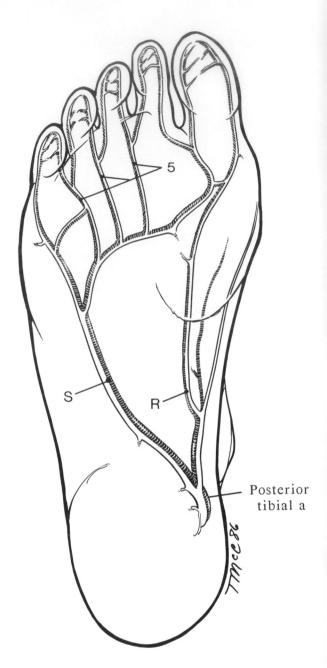

Fig. 15.14  Arterial Supply and
Venous Drainage,
Plantar Surface of Foot

# FOR REVIEW AND THOUGHT

A. Continue your comparison of lower and upper limbs, focusing your attention on leg and foot structures.

Similarities:

Differences:

B. Trace the following structures throughout their course in the limb. Describe their functional significance and important landmarks that might be used to locate them (use Figures 13.3 through 13.5, 14.5 and 14.6, and 15.12 to 15.14). Label Figure 15.15 as a review.

1. Greater and lesser saphenous veins

2. Arterial supply from the pelvis to the foot

3. Tibial nerve

4. Common peroneal nerve

5. Superficial peroneal nerve

6. Deep peroneal nerve

7. Obturator nerve

# CIRCULATORY SYSTEM OUTLINE

## LOWER LIMB

### ARTERIAL

**Bifurcation of the Aorta** - The aorta bifurcates into the common iliac arteries at the level of the body of the fourth lumbar vertebra. The common iliacs split to form external and internal iliac arteries. The external iliac will become the chief supply to the lower limb but several important branches of the internal iliac artery also supply lower limb structures (Figure 14.5).

I. **Internal Iliac**

    A.   **Obturator** - pelvic muscles; hip joint; anterior and medial thigh

    B.   **Superior gluteal** - gluteal muscles

    C.   **Inferior gluteal** - gluteal muscles and posterior thigh

II. **External Iliac**

    D.   **Inferior epigastric**

    E.   **Deep iliac circumflex** - psoas, iliacus, sartorius, tensor fascia latae

III.   **Femoral** (The continuation of the external iliac from inguinal ligament to the adductor hiatus)

    F.   **Superficial and deep external pudendal**

    G.   **Muscular branches** - sartorius, vasti, rectus femoris, adductors

    H.   **Superficial iliac circumflex**

    I.   **Deep femoral (Profunda femoris)**

        1.   Medial femoral circumflex

        2.   Lateral femoral circumflex

    These vessels supply the head and neck of the femur and muscles of the superior third of the thigh.

        3.   Perforating branches - pierce the adductor magnus to supply the posterior thigh

    J.   **Descending genicular** - knee joint

IV. **Popliteal** (The continuation of the femoral from the adductor hiatus to the distal border of the popliteus muscle) (Figure 15.12)

    K.   **Muscular branches** - to adductor magnus and hamstrings

L. **Sural** - gastrocnemius, soleus, plantaris

M. **Superior geniculars (medial and lateral)** - to knee joint proximal to femoral condyles

N. **Inferior geniculars (medial and lateral)** - to knee joint distal to femoral condyles

V. **Anterior Tibial** (One of the terminal branches off the popliteal; courses on the anterior surface of the interosseus membrane to supply the anterior leg musculature) (Figures 15.12, 15.13)

O. **Medial and lateral malleolar branches**

P. **Dorsalis pedis** - to tarsal bones, digital branches to foot, deep plantar arch to sole of foot

    4. Dorsal metatarsal arteries

        a. Proper dorsal digital arteries

VI. **Posterior Tibial** (Other terminal branch of the popliteal; courses on the postero-medial side of the leg) (Figures 15.12, 15.14)

Q. **Peroneal** - deep calf muscles; peroneal muscles

R. **Medial plantar** - medial side of foot and first digit

S. **Lateral plantar** - passes obliquely laterally across the sole to reach the base of the fifth metatarsal, then arches medially and anastomoses with the deep branch of the dorsalis pedis to form the plantar arch

    5. Plantar metatarsal arteries

        b. Proper plantar digital arteries

## VENOUS

The venous drainage of the lower limb is organized much like that of the upper limb. Deep veins (often in pairs) accompany the arteries and have the same names. A system of superficial veins is also present in the lower limb (Figures 15.12, 15.13).

T. Great saphenous vein - originates on the medial side of the dorsal venous arch of the foot and ascends anterior to the medial malleolus, along the medial surface of the leg, passes posterior to the medial tibial and femoral condyles, along the medial surface of the thigh to drain into the femoral vein in the femoral triangle.

U Lesser saphenous vein - begins on the lateral side of the dorsal venous arch of the foot, passes posterior to the lateral malleolus, and ascends the posterior leg to empty into the popliteal vein.

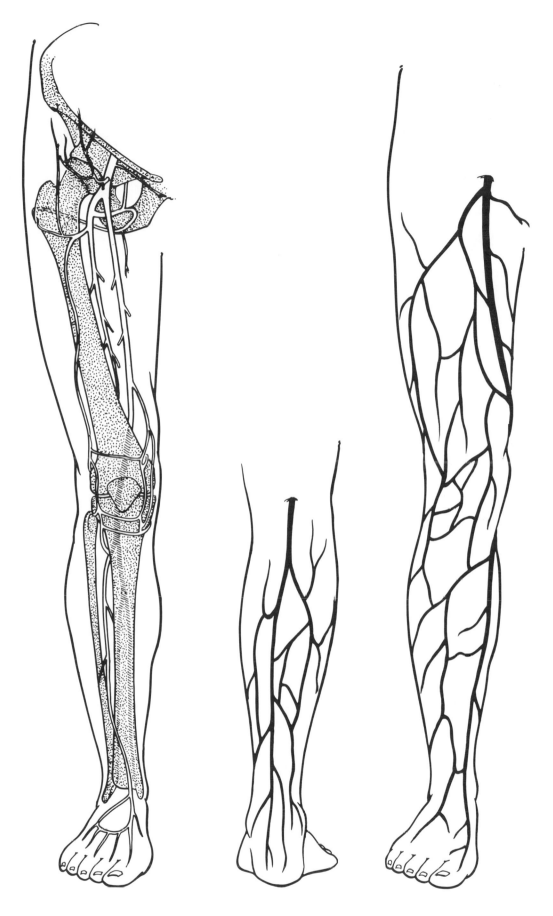

Fig. 15.15  Arteries and Veins of Lower Limb

# NOTES